Praise for
Every Man's Battle

"There is no more common enemy of true manhood than the diversion or the perversion of our sexual capacities. I welcome every contribution to the arsenal of resistance."

—JACK W. HAYFORD, LITT.D., pastor of The Church on the Way
and president of The King's Seminary

"This book will revolutionize the marriage of every man who reads it. Why? Because every man battles sexual temptations and every marriage grows stronger when these temptations are defeated. The vulnerable, honest, and insightful pages of this book reveal what every man must know."

—DRS. LES AND LESLIE PARROTT, authors of *Saving Your Marriage Before It Starts*

"This timely resource presents clear, practical principles for sexual purity. Arterburn and Stoeker call for courage, commitment, and self-discipline as they lead men into a more successful relationship with God, family, and spouse. This book is truly for every man."

—DR. JOHN C. MAXWELL, founder of The INJOY Group

"God has used Steve Arterburn countless times to impact my heart and life; I am thankful for him and his investment in *Every Man's Battle*. I am also grateful for Fred Stoeker. Fred pours himself into this book with honesty, vulnerability, and a practical strategy to fight the good fight. He offers biblical truth and hope to anyone with ears to hear how to battle the war of sexual temptation. Read with an open heart, *Every Man's Battle* may save your marriage and your witness."

—DR. GARY ROSBERG, president of America's Family Coaches and author of *Guard Your Heart* and *The Five Love Needs of Men and Women*

Every Man's Battle

STEPHEN ARTERBURN
FRED STOEKER WITH MIKE YORKEY

Every Man's Battle

Winning the War on Sexual Temptation
One Victory at a Time

WATERBROOK
PRESS

EVERY MAN'S BATTLE
PUBLISHED BY WATERBROOK PRESS
12265 Oracle Boulevard, Suite 200
Colorado Springs, CO 80921

The information on sexual addiction in chapter 3 is drawn from Stephen Arterburn's *Addicted
to "Love"* (Ann Arbor, MI: Vine, 1991), 109–110.

ISBN 978-0-307-45797-4

Published in association with the literary agency of Alive Communications Inc., 7680
Goddard Street, Suite 200, Colorado Springs, CO 80920, ww.alivecommunications.com.

Library of Congress Cataloging-in-Publication Data
Arterburn, Stephen, 1953–
    Every man's battle : winning the war on sexual temptation : one victory at a time / Steve
Arterburn & Fred Stoeker with Mike Yorkey.—1st ed.
        p. cm.
    1. Sex—Religious aspects—Christianity. 2. Temptation. 2. Christian men—Religious life.
I. Stoeker, Fred. II. Yorkey, Mike. III. Title.
    BT708.A77 2000
    241'.66—dc21

                                        00-022845

Printed in the United States of America
2014

10 9

from Stephen Arterburn:

To my friend Jim Burns.

You have displayed great love

and been a premier example of sexual integrity.

————————

from Fred Stoeker:

To my heavenly Father

(thank You that You ran to me);

to my wife, Brenda;

and to my friends Dave Johnson and Les Flanders.

contents

foreword

by Stephen Arterburn

Being part of the Every Man series has been one of the great joys of my life. If I'd written and published only this one series, I would've been completely fulfilled. I owe all this to Fred, who lived out this message long before he was called by God to write about it.

Now, it may sound strange to some, but I believe Fred had one of those rare experiences where God interrupts what we're doing and gives us a new mission. I'm quite confident God spoke to him directly. Fred's coming to me with his manuscript was also part of God's plan, and I'm so glad for it! As a result, my life has been filled with words I could never replace, in the form of e-mails, letters, hugs, crying eyes, and expressions of gratitude. Here are a few comments from the men:

- "Thank you—you've saved my marriage."
- "I am now the man I always wanted to be, living the life I always wanted to live."
- "Oh! This feeling of freedom. I feel so clean!"
- "I don't know where I would be today if it were not for this book."

And from the wives:

- "Thank you for giving the man I married back to me."
- "We would not still be married if not for this book."
- "I wish you could see the man my husband has become today."
- "My man was totally transformed reading your book."

I've received these kinds of messages every day:

I never go into Christian bookstores, but I was jogging one
day and stopped in one. Staring back at me was your book.
I was compelled by it. I ran home, got my money, and
came back and bought it. It changed everything!

Somebody gave me this book about five years ago, and
right before I was about to go back online, there it was
looking up at me from the floor. I picked it up and read
it through my tears. Our marriage has been healed.

Years ago at New Life, we started an Every Man's Battle Workshop
weekend. More than six thousand men have attended since that time. For
a few men, it was just a way to get someone off their backs. But for almost
all, it's been the start of a whole new life. One of my favorite stories is of a
husband who came because his wife demanded it. After the conference he
confessed his affair. He was truly repentant and said he would do anything
to make it up to her. She asked him to sign over all the property and assets
to her—because the name on them wouldn't matter if he was truly finished
with his lust and adultery. She asked him to shave his chest, and she asked
him to get braces on his teeth. He did all three because he realized his
actions had humiliated her and he was willing to do anything to humble
himself and win back her heart. I speak with them both regularly, and they
are doing well.

I'm so glad *you* have come upon this book. For some reason God has
put it in front of you. I'm not just hoping you'll read it; I'm hoping you'll
live it. And while I know personally that every marriage can't be saved, I
know that every man can reclaim his sexual integrity and every spouse can
fully heal. Every man can walk with his head held high—free, honorable,
and a man after God's own heart.

It doesn't really matter what you've done; it's no worse than what others have done. And it doesn't matter where you've been; others have been down that path before. What matters is what you are willing to do now and what you will choose to do. You may have thought you were entitled to do the things you did, but now your entitlement is to live clean, renewed, and without even a hint of impurity. I challenge you to join the millions across this country who have reclaimed their integrity, their faith, and their respect. If Fred and I can do it—those who know us would confirm this— you can certainly do it too.

acknowledgments

I would like to thank Greg Johnson, who introduced me to Fred Stoeker. It was a match made in heaven. And my thanks to Fred, who has brought keen judgment and wisdom to men who are not addicted to sex but who want to be strong with sexual integrity. It has been a privilege working with both of them and with Mike Yorkey and his great writing skills.

—*Stephen Arterburn*

I would like to acknowledge several people who had a profound influence on my life. Mr. Campbell, a talented Vietnam vet in a blue-collar high school, managed to breathe a love of writing into the heart of a jock. Pastors John Palmer and Ray Henderson are my heroes. Joyce Henderson deserves a thank-you for her unflagging support. My mother-in-law, Gwen, was my fiercest defender.

To those who shared their stories and read early versions of the manuscript, thank you. Although I cannot share your names for obvious reasons, you know who you are. You were indispensable. My deepest thanks go to my oldest friends: "Uncle Jim," just remember one thing—you owe me! "Milbie," my respect for you knows no measure. "Hollywood," life is still too precious. R. P., you saw this day coming. And to Dan, Brad, Dick, Gary, Pat, R. B., and Buster, you are the most supportive friends a man could hope for.

And finally, many thanks go to my literary agent, Greg Johnson of Alive Communications, who took a chance on me.

—*Fred Stoeker*

This book is often quite explicit in how the coauthors
describe past struggles—their own and others'—with sexual purity.
For the sake of communicating honestly with readers who face similar
struggles, our goal has been to achieve frankness without causing
offense…thereby making it easier for men to face up
to any uncleanness and to press forward by God's grace and power
into actively sharing His holiness.

four men and this book's story

From editor Mike Yorkey:

I suppose it could be said that every book is an author's labor of love, but this book is a labor of God's love for you, the reader. God has heard a cry from men living in a sexually charged culture, and He has responded by bringing together four men in an unlikely fashion. We feel that the story of how this book arrived in your hands bears an important message to your heart.

I first met Fred Stoeker by telephone back in 1995, while I was editor of *Focus on the Family* magazine. Fred had submitted an article he called "The Art of the Hand-Off," describing how he used Dr. James Dobson's book, *Preparing for Adolescence,* to educate his eleven-year-old son, Jasen, about the birds and the bees. Fred's insightful article arrived in the Focus on the Family mailbags unsolicited; in other words, his submission was one of nearly a thousand that would-be authors sent our way each year, all hoping his or her article would be selected for publication.

Fred didn't know we had room in the magazine for only a dozen unsolicited articles each year. But as I skimmed through Fred's manuscript, something about his first-person story resonated with me, and within a few months we published it.

Sometime later, after I'd moved with my family to San Diego and begun a full-time writing career, Fred sent me a surprise FedEx package. Inside was a thick manuscript. In a cover letter, Fred mentioned that he'd labored evenings, weekends, and months over it, and that he'd already gone through the heart-stopping experience of showing it to his wife, Brenda. She gave the manuscript a thumbs-up, and now Fred needed the opinion of a professional writer and editor. Since I was the only such person he knew, Fred wondered if I wouldn't mind giving it a quick read.

I sat down with Fred's manuscript and was immediately captured by the subject, one that makes most authors beat around the bush. But here was a guy exposing his life story and the life stories of other men. Ogling women. Dreaming about sexual acts with female acquaintances. Sexualized what-ifs and double entendres. Rampant masturbation.

Fred's writing needed structural work and tightening (not unexpectedly, since this was his first manuscript), but beneath the wordiness lay a treasure-trove of truth that could impact a generation of men toward sexual integrity. As I relayed those thoughts to Fred, he asked me to consider rewriting the manuscript for him.

I said yes after more discussion with Fred and prayer, but this wasn't an easy decision. I had just begun a freelance writing career, and choosing the right projects was critical. It's very difficult for first-time authors such as Fred to find a publisher willing to take them on, and I knew his manuscript might never see the light of a publishing day. We plugged ahead, however, trusting God that if He really wanted this message out, He would provide a publisher. WaterBrook Press was God's answer.

From publisher Dan Rich:

When I read Mike and Fred's manuscript, I was immediately struck by its potential. Here was an example of what we at WaterBrook look for most: books that offer Christians encouragement, support, and challenge by authors who can communicate "old truths through new eyes" and lead readers to renewed hope and redemption.

The manuscript could stand on its own, but in our planning sessions we agreed its impact could be much greater if we added the voice of an experienced and widely respected counselor. The perfect fit, we decided, was Steve Arterburn. He had authored or coauthored thirty-five books, had founded a chain of mental-health facilities called the New Life Clinics, and was co-host of the national radio program *New Life Live.*

We asked Steve to come on board and were delighted when he said yes. (In the finished book, the separate contributions of Steve and Fred generally have been blended together with a "we" point of view, except where they narrate specific situations from their own experience and background.)

From coauthor Steve Arterburn:

I eagerly accepted the offer to help shape this book because I believe so much in the topic. In my first phone call to Fred after digging into the manuscript, I told him I believed this book could transform more marriages more deeply than nearly any marriage book I could think of.

How can a book on male sexual purity transform marriages? Because I've found that sexual sins are the termites in the walls and foundations of today's marriages. On my call-in *New Life Live* radio broadcasts, it isn't uncommon to receive several calls each week from men desperate for freedom from impure thought lives and ungodly sexual actions. I'm sure many more men would call if they didn't feel so ashamed.

But I can confidently state that the book you now hold, *Every Man's Battle,* has the potential to free you to love your wife in ways you never dreamed possible.

We've changed the names of people in this book and have even changed a few details of their stories to protect their identities. But their stories are real. They're the stories of pastors, worship leaders, deacons, and elders. They're the stories of white-collar office workers and blue-collar employees. All of them are people who were caught in a terrible snare—just as we once were.

Pursuing sexual integrity, however, is a controversial topic. I've taken heat when I've addressed it on my radio show, and Fred also has received slings and arrows when he's taught or spoken on this subject. We've been ridiculed by the world's sophisticates who find God's standard ridiculous and confining. That's fine with us, because we have a bigger concern—you.

You're in a tough position. You live in a world awash with sensual images available twenty-four hours a day in a variety of mediums: print, television, videos, the Internet—even phones. But God offers you freedom from the slavery of sin through the cross of Christ, and He created your eyes and mind with an ability to be trained and controlled. We simply have to stand up and walk by His power in the right path.

Men need a battle plan, and you'll have one when you finish reading *Every Man's Battle*—a detailed plan for becoming a man of sexual integrity. We've also included a study and discussion guide in the back of the book for your individual use or in a men's group. We believe that *Every Man's Battle* is a great resource for your church's men's retreat.

While Fred and I will be speaking here from the perspective of married men, *Every Man's Battle* isn't just for hitched guys. The principles we describe apply also to the many teens and young adult men who must deal with the issue of sexual integrity while single. Believe us, marriage is no cavalry rescue from sexual temptation, so we've put forth principles to help keep young single men from lusting or developing addictive behavior and to increase their odds of marrying the right person.

While *Every Man's Battle* is directed to men, it can also give women a greater understanding of what men are up against as they battle the age-old problem of the eyes. For that reason, each of the book's six parts concludes with a section called "The Heart of the Woman," based on interviews we conducted with women.

From coauthor Fred Stoeker:

Sexual immorality once held me captive, and after being liberated, I wanted to help other men cleanse themselves from this sin.

After teaching on the topic of male sexual purity in Sunday school, I was approached one day by a man who said, "I always thought that since I was a man I would not be able to control my roving eyes. I didn't know it could be any other way. Now I'm free!" Conversations like that thrilled my heart and confirmed the desire God gave me to help other men out of this quagmire.

As other men approached me and shared their stories of sexual sin, many asked me to write a book. At first, I passed this off as simple complimentary talk. After all, anything I committed to paper had little chance of being published. I'd never written a book before, I wasn't the host of a national radio show, I didn't have a Ph.D., I hadn't studied in seminary.

So why did I start writing a book? Because I felt deeply that if God would grant me such a voice in His kingdom, I could help give even more men some practical steps toward victory and to help set them free to help others.

The following verse inspired me to keep plodding away on this book night after night, month after month:

> Have mercy on me, O God,
>   according to your unfailing love;
> according to your great compassion
>   blot out my transgressions....
> Restore to me the joy of your salvation
>   and grant me a willing spirit, to sustain me.

> *Then I will teach transgressors your ways,*
> *and sinners will turn back to you. (Psalm 51:1,12-13)*

Get it? God's plan is to set sinners free and then use them to teach others. God has been using me in just that way, and I trust He will use you as well.

Are you anxious to get started? Good…so am I. We need real men around here—men of honor and decency, men with their hands where they belong and their eyes and minds focused on Christ. If roving eyes or sexually impure thoughts or even sexual addictions are issues in your life, Steve and I are hoping you'll do something about it.

Isn't it time?

where are we?

our stories

"But among you there must not be even a hint of sexual immorality, or of any kind of impurity" (Ephesians 5:3). If there's a single Bible verse that captures God's standard for sexual purity, this is it.

And it compels this question: In relation to God's standard, is there even a hint of sexual impurity in your life?

For both of us, the answer to that question was yes.

FROM STEVE: COLLISION

In 1983 my wife, Sandy, and I celebrated our first anniversary. One sun-splashed Southern California morning that year, feeling good about life and our future, I hopped in our 1973 Mercedes 450SL—the car of my dreams, white with a black top. I'd owned it for just two months.

I was tooling northbound through Malibu on my way to Oxnard, where I'd been asked to testify in a court hearing about whether a hospital should add an addiction treatment center. I always loved driving along the PCH, as locals called the Pacific Coast Highway. These four lanes of blacktop hugged the golden coastline and provided a close-up view of L.A.'s beach culture. With the top down and the wind blowing in my face, I found that summer morning a good day to be alive.

I never intentionally set out to be girl-watching that day, but I spotted her about two hundred yards ahead and to the left. She was jogging toward me along the coastal sidewalk. From my sheepskin-covered leather seat, I found the view outstanding, even by California's high standards.

My eyes locked on to this goddesslike blonde, rivulets of sweat cascading down her tanned body as she ran at a purposeful pace. Her jogging outfit, if it could be called that in those days before sports bras and spandex, was actually a skimpy bikini. As she approached on my left, two tiny triangles of tie-dyed fabric struggled to contain her ample bosom.

I can't tell you what her face looked like; nothing above the neckline registered with me that morning. My eyes feasted on this banquet of glistening flesh as she passed on my left, and they continued to follow her lithe figure as she continued jogging southbound. Simply by lustful instinct, as if mesmerized by her gait, I turned my head further and further, craning my neck to capture every possible moment for my mental video camera.

Then *blam!*

I might still be marveling at this remarkable specimen of female athleticism if my Mercedes hadn't plowed into a Chevelle that had come to a complete stop in my lane. Fortunately, I was traveling only fifteen miles per hour in the stop-and-go traffic, but the mini-collision crumpled my front bumper and crinkled the hood. And the fellow I smacked into didn't appreciate the considerable damage to his rear end.

I got out of the car—embarrassed, humiliated, saturated with guilt, and unable to offer a satisfying explanation. No way would I tell this guy, "Well, if you'd seen what I saw, you'd understand."

TEN MORE YEARS IN THE DARKNESS

Nor could I tell the truth to my beautiful wife, Sandy. That evening, I put my best spin on the morning's unfortunate event in Malibu. "You see, Sandy, it was stop-and-go, and I was reaching down to change the radio channel, and the next thing I knew I rammed into a Chevy. Lucky no one was hurt."

Actually, my young marriage was hurt—because I was cheating Sandy out of my full devotion, though I didn't know it at the time. Nor was I aware that although I'd vowed to commit my life to Sandy, I hadn't totally committed my eyes to her.

I continued in the darkness for another ten years before realizing I needed to make dramatic changes in the way I looked at women.

FROM FRED: WALL OF SEPARATION

It happened every Sunday morning during our church worship service. I'd look around and see other men with their eyes closed, freely and intensely worshiping the God of the universe. Myself? I sensed only a wall of separation between the Lord and me.

I just wasn't right with God. As a new Christian, I imagined I just didn't know God well enough yet. But nothing changed as time passed.

When I mentioned to my wife, Brenda, that I felt vaguely unworthy of Him, she wasn't the least bit surprised.

"Well, of course!" she exclaimed. "You've never felt worthy to your own father. Every preacher I've known says that a man's relationship with his father tremendously impacts his relationship with his heavenly Father."

"You could be right," I allowed.

I hoped it was that simple. I mulled it over as I recalled my days of youth.

WHAT KIND OF A MAN ARE YOU?

My father, handsome and tough, was a national wrestling champion in college and a bulldog in business. Aching to be like him, I began wrestling in junior high. But the best wrestlers are natural-born killers, and I didn't have a wrestler's heart.

My dad was coaching wrestling at the time at the high school in our small town of Alburnett, Iowa. Though I was still in junior high, he wanted me to wrestle with the older guys, so he brought me to the high-school workouts.

One afternoon we were practicing escapes, and my partner was in the down position. While grappling on the mat, he suddenly needed to blow his nose. He straightened up, pulled his T-shirt to his nose, and violently emptied the contents onto the front of his shirt. We quickly returned to wrestling. As the up man, I was supposed to keep a tight grip on him. Reaching around his belly, my hand slid into his slimy T-shirt. Sickened, I let him go.

Dad, seeing him escape so easily, dressed me down. "What kind of a man are you?" he roared. Staring hard at the mat, I realized that if I had a wrestler's heart, I would have cranked down tightly and ridden out my opponent, maybe grinding his face into the mat in retaliation. But I hadn't.

I still wanted to please Dad, so I tried other sports. At one baseball game, after striking out, I remember hanging my head on the way back to the dugout. "Get your head up!" he hollered for all to hear. I was mortified. Then he wrote me a long letter detailing my every mistake.

Years later, after I'd married Brenda, my father felt she had too much control in our marriage. "Real men take charge of their households," he said.

THE MONSTER

Now, as Brenda and I discussed my relationship with my dad, she suggested I might need counseling. "It surely couldn't hurt," she said.

So I read some books and counseled with my pastor, and my feelings toward Dad improved. But I continued to feel that distance from God during the Sunday morning worship services.

The true reason for that distance slowly dawned on me: There was a hint of sexual immorality in my life. There was a monster lurking about, and it surfaced each Sunday morning when I settled in my comfy La-Z-Boy and opened the Sunday morning newspaper. I would quickly find the department-store inserts and begin paging through the colored newsprint filled with models posing in bras and panties. Always smiling. Always available. I loved lingering over each ad insert. *It's wrong,* I admitted, *but it's such a small thing.* It was a far cry from *Playboy,* I told myself.

I peered through the panties, fantasizing. Occasionally, a model reminded me of a girl I once knew, and my mind rekindled the memories of our times together. I rather enjoyed my Sunday mornings with the newspaper.

As I examined myself more closely, I found I had more than a hint of sexual immorality. Even my sense of humor reflected it. Sometimes a person's innocent phrase—even from our pastor—struck me with a double sexual meaning. I would chuckle, but I felt uneasy.

Why do these double entendres come to my mind so easily? Should a Christian mind create them so nimbly?

I remembered that the Bible said that such things shouldn't even be mentioned among the saints. *I'm worse...I even laugh at them!*

And my eyes? They were ravenous heat-seekers searching the horizon, locking on any target with sensual heat. Young mothers leaning over in shorts to pull children out of car seats. Soloists with silky shirts. Summer dresses with décolletage.

My mind, too, ran wherever it willed. This had begun in my childhood, when I found *Playboy* magazines under Dad's bed. He also subscribed to *From Sex to Sexty,* a publication filled with jokes and comic strips with sexual themes. When Dad divorced Mom and moved to his "bachelor's pad," he hung a giant velvet nude in his living room, overlooking us as we played cards on my Sunday afternoon visits.

Dad gave me a list of chores around his place when I was there. Once I came across a nude photo of his mistress. On another occasion I found an eight-inch ceramic dildo, which he obviously used in his kinky "sex games."

HOPE FOR THE HOPELESS

All this sexual stuff churned deep inside me, destroying a purity that wouldn't return for many years. Settling into college, I soon found myself drowning in pornography. I actually memorized the dates when my favorite soft-core porn magazines arrived at the local drugstore. I especially loved the "Girls Next Door" section of *Gallery* magazine, featuring pictures of nude girls taken by their boyfriends and submitted to the magazine.

Far from home and without any Christian underpinnings, I descended by small steps into a sexual pit. The first time I had sexual intercourse, it was with a girl I *knew* I would marry. The next time, it was with a girl I *thought* I would marry. The time after that, it was with a good friend that I *might* learn to love. Then it was with a female I barely knew who simply wanted to see what sex was like. Eventually, I had sex with anyone at any time.

After five years in California, I found myself with four "steady" girlfriends simultaneously. I was sleeping with three of them and was essentially engaged to marry two of them. None knew of the others. (These days, in my class for premarital couples, I often ask the women what they would think of a man with two fiancées. My favorite response: "He's a hopeless pig!" And I *was* hopeless, living in a pigsty.)

Why do I share all this?

First, so you'll know that I understand what it's like to be sexually ensnared in a deep pit. Second, I want to provide you with hope. As you'll soon see, God worked with me and lifted me out of that pit.

If there's even a hint of sexual immorality in your life, He will work with you as well.

paying the price

FROM FRED: KNOWING WHO TO CALL

Despite the deepening pit I occupied in my single days, I didn't notice anything wrong with my life. Oh, sure, I attended church sporadically, and from time to time the pastor's words penetrated my heart. But who was he? Besides, I loved my girlfriends. *No one's getting hurt,* I reasoned.

My dad had eventually remarried, and when I visited back home in Iowa, my stepmother occasionally dragged me across the river to the Moline Gospel Temple in Moline, Illinois. The gospel was clearly preached, but to me the whole scene was clearly ludicrous. I often laughed cynically. *Those people are crazy!*

After graduating from Stanford University with an honors degree in sociology, I decided to take a job in the San Francisco area as an investment advisor. One spring day in May, I stayed late at the office. Everyone else had gone home, leaving me alone with some troubling thoughts. I swiveled my chair around and propped my feet on the credenza to gaze into a typically grand California sunset.

That evening, as the sun dipped beneath the horizon, I suddenly saw in full clarity what I had become. What I saw was hopelessly ugly. Where once I was blind, now I could see. Instantly, I saw my deep, deep need for a Savior. Because of the Moline Gospel Temple, I knew Whom to call upon.

My prayer that day was born out of the simplicity of a certain heart: "Lord, I'm ready to work with You if You're ready to work with me."

I stood up and walked out of the office, not yet fully realizing what I'd just done. But God knew, and it seemed as if all heaven moved into my life. Within two weeks I had a job back in Iowa and a new life ahead of me. And *no* girlfriends!

FEELING GOOD

Back in Iowa, I began attending a marriage class led by Joel Budd, the associate pastor of my new church. It wasn't long before I realized that I knew nothing about treating women properly. Perhaps it was because my mom and dad were divorced, and I never saw a loving relationship modeled at home. More likely, however, it was because of my own selfishness and sexual sin. Everything I knew about women came from one-night stands and casual dating relationships.

I didn't date during that year under Joel's teaching. I might have been the only man in history to attend a married couples' class for a whole year without even having so much as a single date! But just before the twelve-month mark, I prayed this simple prayer: "Lord, I've been in this class for a year and have learned a lot about women, but I'm not sure I've ever seen these things in real life. I've never really known any Christian girls. Please show me a woman who embodies these godly characteristics."

I wasn't asking for a date, girlfriend, or spouse. I just wanted to see these teachings in practice, in real life, that I might understand them better.

God did far more than that. One week later, He introduced me to my future wife, Brenda, and we fell in love.

Out of our commitment to Christ, Brenda and I decided to stay pure before marriage. She was a virgin—and I wished I were. We did kiss, however, and whoa! Our lip smacking was wonderful! It was my first experience of something I would later discover far more deeply: the physically gratifying payoff that comes from obedience to God's sexual standards.

In a song made popular during my senior year in college, the singer mourned about trying to remember how it used to feel when a kiss was something special. The lyrics from the song resonated sadly with me because, at that point in my life, a kiss meant nothing to me. It was a joyless prerequisite on the path to intercourse. Something was deeply wrong.

But now, having cut way back, in my experience with Brenda the simple kiss became thrilling again. To an old sex-hog like me, this was totally unexpected.

As God continued to work in my life, Brenda and I married, honeymooned in Colorado, then settled into a new apartment building on the edge of a cornfield in a Des Moines suburb. *Is this heaven?* I surely thought so.

Time passed, and at first, I was feeling good. While I was once engaged to two women at the same time, I was now happily married to one woman. While I once drowned in pornography, since my wedding day I hadn't purchased a pornographic magazine. Given my track record, this was remarkable.

STOPPING SHORT

I threw myself into my sales career and my leadership roles at church. Then I became a dad. I relished it all, and my Christian image shined brighter and brighter.

By worldly standards, I was doing great. Just one little problem. By God's standard of sexual purity, I wasn't even close to living His vision for marriage. Clearly I'd taken steps toward purity, but I was learning that God's standards were higher than I'd ever imagined and that my Father had higher hopes for me than I had dreamed.

It soon became clear that I'd stopped far short of holiness. There were the ad inserts, the double entendres, the heat-seeking eyes. My mind continued to daydream and fantasize over old girlfriends. These were more than a hint of sexual immorality.

I was paying the price, and the bills were piling up. First, I could never look God in the eye. I could never fully worship Him. Because I dreamed of being with other women, and rather enjoyed mentally recalling past sexual conquests, I knew I was a hypocrite, and I continued feeling distant from God.

People around me disagreed, saying, "Oh, come on! Nobody can control their eyes and mind, for heaven's sakes! God loves you! It must be something else." But I knew differently.

My prayer life was feeble. Once my son was very sick and had to be rushed to the emergency room. Did I rush into prayer? No, I could only rush others to pray for me. "Have you called our pastor to pray?" I asked Brenda. "Have you called Ron? Have you called Red to pray?" I had no faith in my own prayers because of my sin.

My faith was weak in other ways as well. As a full-commission salesperson, if I lost a number of deals in a row to the competition, I could never be sure if those setbacks weren't somehow caused by my sin. I had no peace.

I was paying a price for my sin.

My marriage was suffering as well. Because of my sin, I couldn't commit 100 percent to Brenda out of fear that she might dump me later. That cost Brenda in closeness. But that's not all. Brenda told me she was experiencing frightening dreams in which she was being chased by Satan. Was my immorality causing spiritual protection to be taken away from her?

My wife was paying a price.

At church, I was an empty suit. I came to church desperately needing ministry and forgiveness. I never arrived ready to minister to others. Of course my prayers were no more effective in God's house than anywhere else.

My church was paying a price.

I remember listening to one sermon in which the pastor talked about "generational sin"—patterns of sin passed from father to son (Exodus 34:7). Sitting in my pew, I recalled that my grandfather had run off from his wife in the middle of the Great Depression, leaving her with six kids to raise. My father left his family to pursue multiple sexual affairs. That same pattern had been passed to me, proven by my own multiple affairs in college. Though saved, I now found that I still didn't have this purity issue settled in my life, and I was scared by the thought of passing this pattern on to my kids.

My children could be paying a price.

I finally made the connection between my sexual immorality and my distance from God. I was paying hefty fines in every area of my life. Having eliminated the visible adulteries and pornography, I looked pure on the outside to everyone else. But to God, I'd stopped short. I'd merely found a middle ground, somewhere between paganism and obedience to God's standard.

DESPERATION

God desired more for me. He had freed me from the pit, but I'd stopped moving toward Him. Having seen the prices I paid and my distance from God, I decided it was time to move closer.

I expected the journey to be easy. After all, I had decided to eliminate pornography and affairs, and they were gone. I figured I could stop the rest of this sexual junk just as easily.

But I couldn't. Every week I said I wouldn't look at those ad inserts, but every Sunday morning the striking photos compelled me. Every week I'd vow to avoid watching R-rated "sexy" movies when I traveled, but every week I'd fail, sweating out tough battles and always losing. Every time I gazed at some glistening jogger, I'd promise to never do it again. But I always did.

What I'd done was simply trade the pornography of *Playboy* and *Gallery* for the pornography of ad inserts and other magazine ads. The affairs? I'd simply traded the physical liaisons for mental affairs and day-dreams—affairs of the eyes and heart. The sin remained because I'd never really *changed*, never rejected sexual sin, never escaped sexual slavery. I'd merely exchanged masters.

A couple of months slipped by, then a couple of years. The distance from God grew wider, the bills stacked higher, and my impurity still ruled me. My faith waned further with each failure. Each desperate loss caused more desperation. While I could always say no, I could never *mean* no.

Something was gripping me, something relentless, something mean.

Like Steve, I eventually found total freedom. Since then, both Steve and I have had the chance to talk to men ensnared in sensual pits. Trapped and desperate to be free, their stories grip the heart. Now that you've heard my story, maybe you'll relate to the men in these next few pages as well.

addiction? or something else?

Before men experience victory over sexual sin, they're hurting and confused. *Why can't I win at this?* they think. As the fight wears on and the losses pile higher, we begin to doubt everything about ourselves, even our salvation. At best, we think that we're deeply flawed. At worst, evil persons. We feel very alone, since men speak little of these things.

But we're *not* alone. Many men have fallen into their own sexual pits.

FROM FRED: ARE YOU NOTICING?

These pitfalls happen easily since much of the sexual immorality in our society is so subtle we sometimes don't recognize it for what it is.

One day a fellow named Mike was telling me about renting the video *Forrest Gump*. "Boy, it was great!" he exclaimed. "Tom Hanks was brilliant. I laughed and cried all the way through it. I know you and Brenda rent good movies for your kids. You should get this one. It was really clean and wholesome."

"No, we won't be bringing *Forrest Gump* into our living room," I responded.

Taken aback, Mike asked, "Why? It was great movie!"

"Well, do you remember that scene at the beginning where Sally Field has sex with the principal to get her son into the 'right' school?"

"Uh…"

"And how about the bare breasts at the New Year's party? The nude on-stage guitar performance? And in the end, when Forrest finally 'got the girl' in the sex scene, she conceived a child out of wedlock. These aren't the types of things I want my kids to see!"

Mike slumped into a chair. "I guess I've been watching movies for so long that I didn't even notice those things."

Are you noticing? Think about it. Suppose you drop your kids at Grandma's for the weekend and decide to watch *Forrest Gump* with your wife. You rent the video, pop some corn, put your arm around your wife, and hit "play." After much laughter and tears, you both agree that *Forrest Gump* was a great movie.

But you got more than entertainment, didn't you? Remember the grunting and panting between Sally Field and the principal? And how, when Sally Field next appeared on screen, you briefly looked her up and down and wondered what it might be like to have her under the sheets? You had your arm around your wife while you were thinking it. Then later, after you retired to bed for a "bit of sport" with your wife, you replaced your wife's face with Sally Field's, and you wondered why she couldn't make you grunt and pant like the principal.

"Come on!" you reply. "This stuff happens all the time." Could be, but listen to these troubling words from Jesus: "I tell you that anyone who looks at a woman lustfully has already committed adultery with her in his heart" (Matthew 5:28).

In light of this Scripture, piddling things like objecting to *Forrest Gump* may not be minor, legalistic meddling. Such subtle influences, added to hundreds of others over time, provide more than a hint of sexual immorality in our lives. Soon, the effect isn't so subtle anymore and not so fun.

STRUGGLES ALL AROUND

Let us share some other stories with you.

Thad is recovering from drug dependency at a local Christian ministry. "I've been trying hard to get my life in order," he told us. "At the drug center, I've learned more about myself and my addiction to drugs. I expected that, since that's why I went there. But I've discovered a second, unexpected thing: I have a problem with lust and impurity.

"I *want* to be free, but I'm becoming frustrated and angry with the church. The Bible says that women should dress modestly, but they don't. The women soloists are always wearing the latest, tightest fashions. I look at them, but all I see are curves and legs. You know, that one who always wears the slit way up the thigh? That thigh flashes with every step she takes. I just get enraged! Why do they make it worse?"

Howard, a Sunday-school teacher, described a life-twisting event in junior high. "I was walking home, and Billy and I stopped by the store to pick up something to drink. I didn't really like Billy, but I felt sorry for him. He didn't have many friends, and he was trying so hard to make some. On the way to the store, he told me about something called masturbation. I'd never heard that word, and he explained what it was. He said all the guys had been experimenting.

"I couldn't get what he told me out of my mind, so that night I tried it. I haven't gone more than a week without masturbating for over fifteen years now!

"I always thought marriage would take the desire away, but it isn't any better, and I'm so ashamed. Not so much by the act itself, but by the things I think about and the movies I watch while doing it. I *know* it's adulterous."

Joe told us he loves women's beach volleyball. "At night, I've had shockingly vivid dreams with these women," he confided. "Some have been so exhilarating and so real that I wake up the next morning *certain* that I've been in bed with them. Heavy with guilt, I wonder where my wife is, sure she has left me over this affair and wondering how I could have done such a thing. Finally, as the cobwebs clear, it slowly dawns on me that it *was* just a dream. But even then I feel uneasy. You want to know why? Because while I know it was just a dream, I'm not at all certain it *wasn't* some form of adultery."

Wally, a businessman and frequent traveler, told us he absolutely dreads hotels. "I always eat a long, leisurely supper," he says, "stalling before returning to my room because I know what's coming. Before too long, I have the TV remote in my hand. I tell myself it'll only be for a minute, but I know I'm lying. I know what I really want. I'm hoping to catch a little sex scene or two as I search the channels. I tell myself that I'll only watch for a while, or that I'll stop before I get carried away. Then my motor gets going and I lust for more, sometimes even turning to the X-rated channel.

"The RPMs are going so high I have to do something, or it feels like my engine will blow. So I masturbate. On a few occasions I fight it, but if I do, later on when I turn the lights out, I'm flooded with lustful thoughts and desires. I stare wide-eyed at the ceiling. I see nothing, but I literally feel the bombardment, the throbbing desire. I have no way to get to sleep, and it's killing me. So I say, 'Okay, if I masturbate, I'll have peace, and I can finally get to sleep.' So I do and guess what? The guilt is so strong I *still* can't get to sleep. I wake up totally exhausted in the morning.

"What's wrong with me? Do other men have this problem? I'm afraid to ask, really. What if this *isn't* how everyone else is? What would that say about *me*? Worse, what if this is how everyone else is? What would that say about the church?"

John wakes up early to watch those morning exercise shows, though he doesn't care much about fitness. "The truth is," he began, "I feel absolutely *compelled* to watch, to catch the closeups of the buttocks, breasts, and especially the inner thighs, and I lust and lust and lust. I sometimes wonder if the producers doing those closeups are just trying to hook men into watching their shows.

"Every day I tell myself that this will be the last time. But by next morning, I'm right there at the TV again."

These men are not weirdos but your next-door neighbors, your fellow workers—even your in-laws. They are you. They are Sunday-school teachers, ushers, deacons. Even pastors aren't immune. One young pastor tearfully detailed to us his ministry and his desire to serve God, expressing in a deeply moving way his devotion to his call. But his tears turned to wrenching sobs as he spoke of his bondage to pornography. His spirit was willing, but his flesh was very weak.

SPINNING IN THE CYCLES

What about you? Maybe it's true that when you and a woman reach a door simultaneously, you wait to let her go first, but not out of honor. You want to follow her up the stairs and look her over. Maybe you've driven your rental car to the parking lot of a local gym between appointments, watching scantily clad women bouncing in and out, fantasizing and lusting—even masturbating—in the car. Maybe you can't stay away from Sixth Avenue, where the prostitutes ply their trade. Not that you'd ever hire one. Or maybe you don't buy *Playboy* back home, but when you're on a business trip, you just can't help yourself.

You're still teaching Sunday school, still singing in the choir, still supporting your family. You've been faithful to your wife…well, at least you haven't had an actual, physical affair. You're getting ahead, living in a nice home with nice cars and nice clothes and a nice future. *People look to me as an example,* you reason. *I'm okay.*

Yet privately, your conscience dims until you can't quite tell what's right or wrong anymore, watching things like *Forrest Gump* without even noticing the sexuality. You're choking in the sexual prison you've made, wondering where the promises of God have gone. You spin in the same sinful cycles, year after year.

And nagging you is the worship. The prayer times. The distance, always the distance from God.

Meanwhile, your sexual sin remains so consistent that you can set your watch by it.

Rick, for instance, walks down the hall at breaktime just to glance through the glass doors of another office, where a bosomy secretary answers phones and directs clients. "Every day at 9:30, I wave at her and she smiles back," he says wistfully. "She's beautiful, and her clothes—let's just say they really accentuate her best features. I don't know her name, but I'm actually depressed when she's absent from work."

Similarly, Sid races home by 4 P.M. every summer day. That's when his neighbor Angela sunbathes right outside his window. "At four o'clock, she lies out in a bikini, and she doesn't know I can see her. I can gaze to my heart's content. She's so sexy I can hardly stand it, and I masturbate every day I see her."

Take This Test

Are these men addicted? The compelling sexual cravings are certainly strong evidence.

Here's a little test you can take. You don't need a pencil; you just need to be honest with yourself. Answer yes or no to the following questions:

1. Do you lock on when an attractive woman comes near you?
2. Do you masturbate to images of other women?

3. Have you found your wife to be less sexually satisfying?

4. Are you holding a grudge against your wife—a grudge that gives you a sense of entitlement?

5. Do you seek out sexually arousing articles or photo spreads in newspapers or magazines?

6. Do you have a private place or secret compartment that you keep hidden from your wife?

7. Do you look forward to going away on a business trip?

8. Do you have behaviors that you can't share with your wife?

9. Do you frequent porn-related sites on the Internet?

10. Do you watch R-rated movies, sexy videos, or the steamy VH1 channel for gratification?

If you've answered yes to any of these questions, you're lurking at the door of sexual addiction. You're *inside* that door if you can answer yes to the following questions:

1. Do you watch pay-per-view sexually explicit TV channels at home or on the road?

2. Do you purchase pornography on the Internet?

3. Do you rent adult movies?

4. Do you watch nude dancing?

5. Do you call 900-numbers to have phone sex?

6. Do you practice voyeurism?

If you said yes to the last six questions, you very well could be sexually addicted. When Titus 2:3 admonishes against being "addicted to much wine," the Greek word used for "addicted" means to be brought into bondage, much like a slave. If you think you're a slave to your sexual passions, then you need to get help for your addiction by talking to a counselor or therapist. (You can call toll-free 1-800-NEW-LIFE (639-5433) and ask about treatment options. One option is a program for sex addiction called the "New Liberty Program.")

FROM STEVE: STRONG APPETITE OR ADDICTION?

Before we go further, I need to make the point that it's easy to confuse normal sexual desire and conduct with addictive compulsions and gratification. A person can have a stronger-than-normal sexual appetite and not be a sex addict.

I wrote about the characteristics of addictive sex in my book *Addicted to "Love."* These characteristics are summarized below. Read the list to help you distinguish between addictive sex and a stronger-than-normal sexual appetite:

- *Addictive sex is done in isolation and is devoid of relationship.* This doesn't necessarily mean that it's done while physically alone. Rather it means that mentally and emotionally the addict is detached, or isolated, from human relationship and contact. Addictive sex is "mere sex," sex for its own sake, sex divorced from authentic interaction of persons. This is most clear regarding fantasy, pornography, and masturbation. But even regarding sex involving a partner, the partner isn't really a "person" but a cipher, an interchangeable part in an impersonal—almost mechanical— process. The most intimately personal of human behaviors becomes utterly impersonal.

- *Addictive sex is secretive.* In effect, sex addicts develop a double life, practicing masturbation, going to porn shops and massage parlors, all the while hiding what they're doing from others—and in a sense, even from themselves.

- *Addictive sex is devoid of intimacy.* Sex addicts are utterly self-focused. They cannot achieve genuine intimacy because their self-obsession leaves no room for giving to others.

- *Addictive sex is victimizing.* The overwhelming obsession with self-gratification blinds sex addicts to the harmful effects their behavior is having on others and on themselves.

- *Addictive sex ends in despair.* When married couples make love, they're more fulfilled for having had the experience. Addictive sex leaves the participants feeling guilty, regretting the experience. Rather than fulfilling them, it leaves them feeling more empty.
- *Addictive sex is used to escape pain and problems.* The escapist nature of addictive sex is often one of the clearest indicators that it is present.

Like any addiction, sex addiction is progressive. It's like "athlete's foot of the mind," as one person described it. It never goes away. It's always asking to be scratched, promising relief. To scratch, however, is to cause pain and to intensify the itch.

FROM FRED: A THUNDERBOLT

Having "athlete's foot of the mind" was how I felt. I vividly remember my internal struggles between the consequences of my sin and the pleasure of my sin. I remember when those consequences finally got to the point where they weren't worth the pleasure of the sin.

But did I qualify as an "addict"?

When I read one author's description of a four-step addiction cycle—preoccupation, ritualization, compulsive sexual behavior, then despair—I knew I'd lived that pattern. I was certain that what I'd experienced, and what these other men had experienced, was addiction.

But a thunderbolt hit me when the author outlined the three levels of addiction (keep in mind that this wasn't a Christian book):

Level 1: Contains behaviors that are regarded as normal, acceptable, or tolerable. Examples include masturbation, homosexuality, and prostitution.

Level 2: Behaviors that are clearly victimizing and for which legal sanctions are enforced. These are generally seen as nuisance offenses, such as exhibitionism or voyeurism.

Level 3: Behaviors that have grave consequences for the victims and legal consequences for the addicts, such as incest, child molestation, or rape.

Did you read that list closely? Did you notice that the examples of Level 1 include not just masturbation, which most men practice at times, but also homosexuality and prostitution? We would be willing to wager that the vast majority of men reading this book do not engage in homosexual acts or use prostitutes. By the definition above, maybe we aren't addicts after all.

But if we aren't addicts, what are we?

FROM STEVE: "FRACTIONAL ADDICTION"

Before we answer that question, let's think again about those "three levels of addiction" as described above. From our Christian perspective, let's insert another level at the bottom of the addiction scale. If we categorized being *totally* pure and holy as the zero level, most Christian men we know would fall somewhere between Level 0 and Level 1.

If you're one of the many men in this area, it probably isn't at all helpful to label you as an "addict" or to imply that victory will take years of therapy. Instead, victory can be measured in weeks, as we'll describe later.

Your "addictive" behaviors are not rooted in some deep, dark, shadowy mental maze, as they are in Levels 1, 2, and 3. Rather, they're based on pleasure highs. Men receive a chemical high from sexually charged images—a hormone called epinephrine is secreted into the bloodstream, which locks into the memory whatever stimulus is present at the time of the emotional excitement. I've counseled men who became emotionally and sexually stimulated just from entertaining thoughts of sexual activity. A guy dead set on purchasing *Hustler* at his local 7-Eleven is sexually stimulated long before he even steps into the convenience store. His stimulation began in his thought process, which triggered his nervous system, which secreted epinephrine into the bloodstream.

From my counseling experience, I believe it's often true that those men living at Level 1 or worse have deep psychological problems that will take years to work through. But relatively few men live there. Our contention is that the vast majority of men stuck in sexual sin are living between Level 0 and Level 1. We can call this a "fractional addiction" since it represents living at a level that's a fraction between zero and one. When we're fractionally addicted, we surely experience addictive drawings, but we aren't compelled to act to salve some pain. We're compelled by the chemical high and the sexual gratification it brings.

Another way of looking at the scope of the problem is to picture a bell curve. According to our experiences, we figure around 10 percent of men have no sexual-temptation problem with their eyes and their minds. At the other end of the curve, we figure there's another 10 percent of men who are sexual addicts and have a serious problem with lust. They've been so beaten and scarred by emotional events that they simply can't overcome that sin in their lives. They need more counseling and a transforming washing by the Word. The rest of us comprise the middle 80 percent, living in various shades of gray when it comes to sexual sin.

GOING FOR FORBIDDEN FRUIT

As I described earlier, I lived in this area of fractional addiction during my first decade of marriage as well as earlier in my adolescence and college years. My interest in the female body had been formed when I was four and five years old and visiting my grandfather's machine shop in Ranger, Texas. I loved walking into that old shop filled with lathes and presses, where Grandpa made tools to retrieve broken oil-well pipes. His office wall was adorned with nude pinups, and I stared at these voluptuous naked women in awe.

As I grew older, I saw women more as objects than people who had feelings. Pornography became for me an enticement to forbidden love. Many young women I dated in high school and college were sexually pure and stayed sexually pure while we dated, but I was always manipulating and conniving, going for what was forbidden.

I later tasted the forbidden fruit when I entered the promiscuous period of my life. When I did have premarital sex, it gave me a sense of control and ownership, as if these young women belonged to me. They were objects of my gratification, just like those pictures on the wall of my grandfather's shop.

SECRETS

When I met Sandy, we made a commitment not to have sex before we married, and we didn't. I didn't tell her about my past, however, nor did I disclose all the secret compartments named Past Relationships or Promiscuity. As a result, I dragged my past into our marriage, which produced problems, just as she dragged her own set of problems into our marital union. Our marriage almost didn't survive the first few tumultuous years.

The angrier I became at Sandy during those dark times, the more lustful my thoughts would be. I began living in a secret world of gratification that came from looking at other beautiful women, whether they were found in fashion magazines or women's magazines. Looking back, I see how those images broke the connection between us. But I was ignorant—ignorant of the fact that I was hurting my marriage. After all, I wasn't having sex with anyone except her. I wasn't getting all-over massages in seedy parts of town or even masturbating to those photo spreads of barely clad models. But what I *was* doing was bringing something into the marriage that didn't need to be there. I felt entitled to have this secret world where I experienced small doses of gratification by looking up and down at well-built women. That *hurt* my marriage.

What I, along with Fred, needed to do was train my eyes and mind to behave. I needed to align my eyes and mind with Scripture and to avoid every hint of sexual immorality.

Before we get into an action plan for realigning your eyes and mind, however, we need to talk further about the roots of the sexual bondage. How is it that so many Christian men can't find their way out of sexual sin? We'll start exploring why in the next chapter.

The Heart of a Woman

(Male sexual impurity can be unsettling, even shocking, to women, which is why we're including sections from interviews we conducted with women regarding *Every Man's Battle*.)

Deena, when asked for her reaction to this book's premise, replied, "This stuff is crazy. Women don't have that problem!"

Fawn decided men and women are so different in their sexual wiring that it defies understanding. "I was surprised to learn," she said, "that Christian men have this problem even after they're married. I found the intensity of the problem to be shocking."

Cathy said, "I did not know the depth that men would go and the risk they would take to satisfy their desires. I was unaware of how intense these temptations are and how much defense a man must muster to avoid stepping over God's boundaries."

Andrea said that, from talking with her father and the different guys she dated, she knows men are easily attracted visually. But she never realized the major extent of this problem until she met her future husband. "At the time, he was my closest friend in the youth group, but we were not romantically inclined," Andrea said. "He did feel safe enough with me to share his problem with pornography. It was quite a battle for him, as he had first been exposed to it in third grade. I was a little amazed by it all because, although I was attracted to guys by their looks during my dating years, the physical attraction I felt was nothing compared to what a man feels when looking at a woman."

Brenda, Fred's wife, also participated in the interviews. She summarized the typical female response: "I don't want to sound mean, but because women don't generally experience this problem, it seems to us that some men are uncontrolled perverts who don't think about anything but sex. It even affects my trust in men, knowing that pastors and deacons could have this problem. I don't like it that men lustfully take advantage of women in their thoughts, although I realize that women can be largely to blame because of what they wear. It's at least *some* comfort to know that *many* men have this problem. Since most men are affected, we really can't call you guys perverts."

(Gee, thanks Brenda. Actually, you made an important point, and it brings up additional thoughts from a man's perspective. We men understand your shock. After all, we're often overwhelmed in the sexual area, and we loathe it ourselves. That's why we want mercy, although we know we don't *deserve* mercy. How much mercy can be found in a woman's heart when she looks upon this problem? Not surprisingly, it depends upon her husband's situation.)

There's a natural tug-of-war in the hearts of women between pity and disgust, between mercy and judgment.

Ellen said, "After hearing about this, I was surprised that married men would have so much trouble. I feel very sorry for them. When I asked my own husband about it, he was honest with me that he had some struggles, and at first I was hurt. Then I just felt thankful that he would share with me. He hasn't had a major problem in this area, for which I'm thankful."

Cathy leans toward mercy as well. "My husband is regularly bombarded with sexy images, and I was pleased with his honesty regarding that," she said. "I *want* to know the temptations he faces. It will only help me be more sympathetic to his plight. I didn't feel betrayed because he's proven faithful in this battle. Other women are not so lucky."

What about those women whose husbands have been losing big in the battle?

"When my husband and I talked about this, he was honest," Deena conveyed, "and I was *very* angry with him. I was hurt. I felt deeply betrayed because I'd been dieting and working out to keep my weight down so that I would always look nice to him. I couldn't figure out why he still needed to look at other women."

Women told us that they struggle between pity and anger, and their feelings may ebb and flow with the tide of their husband's battle. Let us direct this advice to women reading this book: Though you know you should pray for him and fulfill him sexually, sometimes you won't want to. Talk to each other openly and honestly, then do the right thing.

PART II

how we got here

mixing standards

For most of us, becoming ensnared by sexual sin happened easily and naturally, like slipping off an icy log. Why is that?

As we'll see later, our maleness brings us a natural vulnerability to sexual sin. But for now let's explore how the fickle human heart makes us vulnerable as well.

Perhaps you've mustered the hope that you would someday be free from sexual sin and expected to grow out of it as naturally as you grew into it—like outgrowing acne. Perhaps you waited with each birthday for your sexual impurity to clear up. It never did. Later you assumed you'd be freed naturally through marriage. But—as for many of us—that didn't happen either.

FROM FRED: MISPLACED CONFIDENCE

When Mark signed up for my premarriage class, he told me, "The whole problem of impurity has been a mess. I've been hooked for years, and I'm counting on marriage to free me. I'll be able to have sex whenever I want it. Satan won't be able to tempt me at all!"

When we got together a few years later, I wasn't surprised to hear that marriage hadn't fixed the problem. "You know, Fred, my wife doesn't desire sex as often as I do," he said.

Oh, really?

"I don't want to seem like a sex addict or anything, but I probably have as many unmet desires now as I did before marriage. On top of all that, some areas of sexual exploration seem embarrassing or immodest to her. Sometimes she even calls them 'kinky.' I think she's rather prudish, but what do I say?"

In our experience, not much!

MARRIAGE: NO SEXUAL NIRVANA

That marriage doesn't eliminate sexual impurity comes as no surprise to married men, although it does for teens and young singles. Ron, a youth pastor in Minnesota, said that when he challenges young men to be sexually pure, their response is, "That's easy for you to say, Pastor. You're married! You can have sex anytime you want!" Young singles believe that marriage creates a state of sexual nirvana.

If only it were so. First of all, sex has different meanings to men and women. Men primarily receive intimacy just before and during intercourse. Women gain intimacy through touching, sharing, hugging, and communication. Is it any wonder that the frequency of sex is less important to women than to men, as Mark woefully discovered? Because of the differences between men and women, forming a satisfying sex life in marriage is hardly a slam dunk. It's more like making a half-court shot.

Second, life throws hard curves. Lance married his sweetheart only to find that his wife had a structural deficiency that made intercourse very painful. It took surgery and months of rehabilitation to correct the problem. For Bill, his wife once became so ill that he couldn't have intercourse for eight months. Did these circumstances free Lance and Bill to say, "God, I'll just keep using pornography until You heal my wife"? We don't think so.

Third, your wife may suddenly become much different from the woman you courted. Larry, a strapping, handsome young pastor in Washington, D.C., has a great Christian heritage. His father is a wonderful pastor, and Larry was thrilled when God also called him into the ministry. When Larry met Linda, a striking blond bombshell, they appeared meant for each other, a regular Ken and Barbie set.

After their wedding day, however, Larry found Linda to be far more interested in her career than in fulfilling him sexually. Not only was she disinterested in sex, she often used it as a manipulative weapon to get her own way. Consequently, Larry doesn't have sex very often. Twice a month is a bonanza, and once every two months is the norm. What's Larry supposed to say to God? *Lord, Linda is being ungodly! Change her, and then I'll stop masturbating!* Hardly. Marriage didn't satisfy Larry's sexual needs, but God still expects purity.

Your purity must not depend upon your mate's health or desire. God holds *you* responsible, and if you don't gain control before your wedding day, you can expect it to crop up after the honeymoon. If you're single and watching sensual R-rated movies, wedded bliss won't change this habit. If your eyes lock on passing babes, they'll still roam after you say "I do." You're masturbating now? Putting that ring on your finger won't keep your hands off yourself.

WHAT'S GOING ON HERE?

When marriage doesn't immediately solve our problem, we cling to the hope that, given enough time, marriage may yet free us. Andy told us, "I once read that a man's sex drive drops in his thirties and forties, while a woman's sex drive reaches its peak during that time. For a while, I thought that Jill and I would meet in some blissful middle ground. It didn't happen."

But freedom from sexual sin rarely comes through marriage or the passage of time. (The phrase "dirty old man" should tell us something about that.) So if you're tired of sexual impurity and of the mediocre, distant relationship with God that results from it, quit waiting for marriage or some hormone drop to save the day.

If you want to change, recognize that you're impure because you've diluted God's standard of sexual purity with your own. That's the first of three reasons we'll look at for how easily men fall into sexual sin.

We've said earlier that God's standard is that we avoid every hint of sexual immorality in our lives. If we followed this standard, we would never see sexual bondage. So we *should* be amazed that so many Christian men are under that bondage.

Our heavenly Father is amazed. Here's our paraphrase of some questions God asked (in Hosea 8:5-6) that reveal His amazement:

> What is going on here? Why are my children choosing to
> be impure? They are Christians, for heaven's sakes! When
> are they going to start acting like it?

God knows we're Christians and that we can choose to be pure. So why don't we?

We aren't victims of some vast conspiracy to ensnare us sexually; we've simply chosen to mix in our own standards of sexual conduct with God's standard. Since we found God's standard too difficult, we created a mixture—something new, something comfortable, something mediocre.

What do we mean by "mixture"? Perhaps a good example is the muddled definition of "sexual relations" that surfaced in the sex scandal involving President Bill Clinton. After the president stated under oath that he did not have sexual relations with Monica Lewinsky, he later explained that he didn't view oral sex as being in that category. So by that definition, he hadn't committed adultery.

That represents quite a contrast to the standard Christ taught: "But I tell you that anyone who looks at a woman lustfully has already committed adultery with her in his heart" (Matthew 5:28).

NAIVE, REBELLIOUS, CARELESS

Why do we so easily mix in our own standards with God's? Why are we so soft in our choices regarding sexual sin?

Sometimes we're simply naive. Do you remember seeing the animated Disney classic *Pinocchio* when you were growing up? Pinocchio knew it was the right thing for all little boys to go to school. On his way there, however, he met some scoundrels who painted a wonderful picture of spending the day at a place called Adventure Island, a sort of amusement park just offshore. They gave Pinocchio a free ticket on the ferry over, but he didn't know that at day's end all the boys would be turned into donkeys and be sold to pull carts in the coal mines for the rest of their lives. Likewise, we can be naive and foolish regarding God's standard for sexual purity as we stumble blindly into wrong "because everyone else is doing it."

But sometimes we choose wrong sexual standards not because we're naive, but simply because we're rebellious. We're like Lampwick, a swaggering boy who takes the lead in diverting Pinocchio to Adventure Island. Lampwick comes across as distasteful from the moment he appears on the screen with his macho posturing, spitting, and sneering little voice. You ask yourself, *Where are his parents? Why don't they do something?* You know he's fully aware of the evil he's doing. Whatever the aftermath, he richly deserves it.

Perhaps, with a rebelliousness like Lampwick's, you know sexual immorality is wrong but you do it anyway. You love your trips to Adventure Island, despite the hidden price you pay at the end of the day.

Or maybe you've considered God's standard too ridiculous to take seriously. In one singles Bible study group, the discussion turned to sexual purity. Many had been married before and were struggling with loneliness. When someone suggested that God expects even singles to avoid every hint of sexual immorality, one attractive young woman blurted out, "Nobody could possibly expect us to live that way!" The rest of the group heartily agreed with her, except for two who defended God's standard.

DESTRUCTION AND LOATHING

Whether you've been naive, rebellious, or foolishly negligent in taking God's standard seriously, mixing in your own standards leads to being ensnared and even worse.

Mixture can destroy a people. When the Israelites left Egypt and were led to the Promised Land, God told them to cross the Jordan River and destroy every evil thing in their new homeland. That meant killing all the heathen people and crushing their gods to powder. God warned them that if they failed to do this, their culture would "mix" with the pagans and they would adopt their depraved practices.

But the Israelites were not careful to destroy everything. They found it easier and easier to stop short. In time, the things and people left undestroyed became a snare. The Israelites became adulterous in their relationship to God and repeatedly turned their backs on Him.

As promised, He removed them from their land. But just before the destruction of Jerusalem and the final deportation of her inhabitants, God prophesied this about His people in their coming captivity:

> Then in the nations where they have been carried captive,
> those who escape will remember me—how I have been grieved
> by their adulterous hearts, which have turned away from me,
> and by their eyes, which have lusted after their idols. They will
> *loathe themselves* for the evil they have done. (Ezekiel 6:9)

When we entered the Promised Land of our salvation, we were told to eliminate every hint of sexual immorality in our lives. Since entering that land, have you failed to crush sexual sin? Every hint of it? If not, have you come to the point of loathing yourself for that failure? If that's where you are, there's hope for you.

God's Standard from the Bible

Because our own standards on sexual purity have been so mixed with God's, and since many Christians don't read their Bibles very often, many men have no clue about God's standard for sexual purity.

Did you know that we're commanded to avoid sexual impurity in nearly every book of the New Testament? The following is a selection of passages that teach God's concern for our sexual purity. (High-lighted in italics are key words indicating what we're to avoid in the sexual realm):

> But I [Jesus] tell you that anyone who *looks at a woman lustfully* has already committed adultery with her in his heart. (Matthew 5:28)

> For from within, out of men's hearts, come evil thoughts, *sexual immorality,* theft, murder, *adultery,* greed, malice, deceit, *lewdness,* envy, slander, arrogance and folly. All these evils come from inside and make a man "unclean." (Mark 7:21-23)

> You are to abstain from...*sexual immorality.* (Acts 15:29)

> So let us put aside the deeds of darkness and put on the armor of light. Let us behave decently, as in the daytime, not in *orgies* and drunkenness, not in *sexual immorality* and *debauchery,* not in dissension and jealousy. (Romans 13:12-13)

> I am writing you that you must not associate with anyone who calls himself a brother but is *sexually immoral* or greedy, an idolater

or a slanderer, a drunkard or a swindler. With such a man do not even eat. (1 Corinthians 5:11)

The body is not meant for *sexual immorality,* but for the Lord. (1 Corinthians 6:13)

Flee from *sexual immorality.* (1 Corinthians 6:18)

I am afraid that when I come again...I will be grieved over many who have sinned earlier and have not repented of the *impurity, sexual sin* and *debauchery* in which they have indulged. (2 Corinthians 12:21)

So I say, live by the Spirit, and you will not gratify the desires of the sinful nature.... The acts of the sinful nature are obvious: *sexual immorality, impurity* and *debauchery.* (Galatians 5:16,19)

But among you there must not be even a hint of *sexual immorality,* or of any kind of *impurity,* or of greed, because these are improper for God's holy people. Nor should there be obscenity, foolish talk or coarse joking, which are out of place. (Ephesians 5:3-4)

Put to death, therefore, whatever belongs to your earthly nature: *sexual immorality, impurity, lust, evil desires* and greed, which is idolatry. Because of these, the wrath of God is coming. (Colossians 3:5-6)

It is God's will that you should be sanctified: that you should avoid *sexual immorality;* that each of you should learn to control his own body in a way that is holy and honorable, not in *passionate lust* like the heathen, who do not know God.... For God did not call us to be *impure,* but to live a holy life. (1 Thessalonians 4:3-5,7)

See that no one is *sexually immoral*. (Hebrews 12:16)

Marriage should be honored by all, and the marriage bed kept pure, for God will judge the adulterer and all the *sexually immoral*. (Hebrews 13:4)

For you have spent enough time in the past doing what pagans choose to do—living in *debauchery, lust,* drunkenness, *orgies,* carousing and detestable idolatry. (1 Peter 4:3)

In a similar way, Sodom and Gomorrah and the surrounding towns gave themselves up to *sexual immorality* and perversion. They serve as an example of those who suffer the punishment of eternal fire. (Jude 7)

Nevertheless, I [Jesus] have a few things against you: You have people there who hold to the teaching of Balaam, who taught Balak to entice the Israelites to sin...by committing *sexual immorality*. (Revelation 2:14)

Nevertheless, I [Jesus] have this against you: You tolerate that woman Jezebel, who calls herself a prophetess. By her teaching she misleads my servants into *sexual immorality*. (Revelation 2:20)

But the cowardly, the unbelieving, the vile, the murderers, the *sexually immoral,* those who practice magic arts, the idolaters and all liars—their place will be in the fiery lake of burning sulfur. This is the second death. (Revelation 21:8)

Isn't that something? More than half of the books in the New Testament are represented here.

Drawing from these passages, let's summarize God's standard for sexual purity:

- Sexual immorality begins with the lustful attitudes of our sinful natures. It is rooted in the darkness within us. Therefore sexual immorality, like other sins that enslave unbelievers, will incur God's wrath.

- Our bodies were not meant for sexual immorality, but for the Lord, who has both created us and called us to live in sexual purity. His will is that every Christian be sexually pure—in his thoughts and his words as well as in his actions.

- Therefore it is holy and honorable to completely avoid sexual immorality—to repent of it, to flee from it, and to put it to death in our lives, as we live by the Spirit. We've spent enough time living like pagans in passionate lust.

- We should not be in close association with another Christian who persists in sexual immorality.

- If you entice others to sexual immorality (maybe in the backseat or back room), Jesus Himself has something against you!

Clearly, God *does* expect us to live according to His standard. In fact, in 1 Thessalonians 4:3 the Bible flatly states that this is God's will.

So take His command seriously—*Flee sexual immorality!*

obedience or mere excellence?

Why do we find it so easy to mix our standards of sexual sin and so difficult to firmly commit to true purity?

Because we're used to it. We easily tolerate mixed standards of sexual purity because we tolerate mixed standards in most other areas of life.

EXCELLENCE OR OBEDIENCE?

Question: What's your aim in life—excellence or obedience?

What's the difference? To aim for obedience is to aim for perfection, not for "excellence," which is actually something less.

"Wait a minute!" you reply. "I thought excellence and perfection were the same thing."

Sometimes they appear to be. But mere excellence allows room for a mixture. In most arenas, excellence is not a fixed standard at all. It's a mixed standard.

Let us show you what we mean. American businesses are in search of excellence. They could be in search of perfection, of course—perfect products, perfect service—but perfection is too costly and eats into profits. Rather than be perfect, businesses know it's enough to *seem* perfect to their customers. By stopping short of perfection, they find a profitable balance between quality and costs.

To find this balance, they often look to their peers to discover the "best practices" of their industry: *How far can we go and still seem perfect? By how far can we stop short?* Businesses find it profitable to stop short at the middle ground of excellence because perfection costs too much.

But is it profitable for Christians to stop short at the middle ground of excellence where costs are low, balanced somewhere between paganism and obedience? Not at all! While in business it's profitable to *seem* perfect, in the spiritual realm it's merely *comfortable* to seem perfect. It is never profitable.

Clearly, excellence isn't the same as obedience or perfection. The search for excellence leaves us overwhelmingly vulnerable to snare after snare since it allows room for mixture. The search for obedience or perfection does not.

Excellence is a *mixed* standard, while obedience is a *fixed* standard. We want to shoot for the fixed standard.

From Fred: Asking the Wrong Question

I was the perfect example of someone who wasn't shooting for God's fixed standard of obedience. I was teaching classes at church, chairing activities groups, and attending discipleship classes. My church attendance was exemplary, and I spoke the Christian language. Like the businessman seeking the best business practices, I was asking myself, *How far can I go and still be called a Christian?* The question I should have been asking was, *How holy can I be?*

Let me demonstrate the difference between excellence and obedience through a couple of stories from my premarriage class. When each seven-week session begins, I ask the students what they desire in marriage. During a recent class, all six couples declared that they wanted to build their relationships upon God's principles. Then I asked this question: Is it all right to modify the truth to avoid unpleasantness in the home?

Each answered no, unanimously agreeing that modifying the truth was lying and that none of them would do that in *their* homes.

"Really?" I asked. "Then what about this? Brenda has had four children, and through the years her weight has slid between four different wardrobe sizes. [Much laughter usually follows this comment.] During transitions between sizes, she often hoped to wear something from the smaller-size wardrobe to church. Squeezing into it, she'd ask me, 'Is this too tight?' She wanted to know whether the dress fit or whether it would draw attention to her weight. Often it was a close call, and I would have to choose between modifying the truth or hurting her feelings and discouraging her.

"Was it okay for me to modify the truth to avoid this unpleasantness? It's a small thing, after all, and I love her. If I told the truth, it would hurt her feelings, and I don't like to hurt her feelings.

"What would you do? Would you modify the truth?"

Amazingly, only moments after declaring that they would never modify the truth in their home, five out of the six couples now said they *would* indeed modify the truth to avoid this particular unpleasantness.

They can speak the Christian language, and they certainly sound excellent. But can they *live* Christian truth?

With excellence we try to cover our disobedient tracks. Pete and Mary attended my premarriage class, and Pete impressed me from day one. He lapped up anything I said, nodding in assent at even the most difficult teachings regarding the husband's responsibilities (such as servanthood).

At the end of the seventh week, Pete and Mary stopped me after class. "Your discussion on sexual purity really hit home last week," Pete began, "especially when you said that viewing pornography and X-rated movies won't strengthen your sex life. My first wife used to rent X-rated movies for me, and we would watch them together before going to bed. In the end, it hurt us." Then he added, "Mary and I will not do this in our marriage." So far, so good.

But Mary, stepping in, said, "We've been having an ongoing struggle over what we watch together. We'll often rent a movie to watch at my apartment, but you know how it is. Most of the popular movies have some pretty racy scenes, and I'm feeling more and more uncomfortable with this. When it gets steamy, I tell Pete we need to turn it off, but he gets angry, arguing that we've invested good money in the rental and it's a waste of money to shut it off. So I go off into the kitchen to do some work while he finishes watching."

She got a tear in her eye and looked down. "I don't feel these movies are good for us," she said. "I've asked him to stop for my sake, but he won't. We make it a practice to pray together before he goes home, but after these movies, I often feel dirty and cheap. I feel these movies are coming between us."

Of course, Pete was embarrassed. Was he in search of excellence or obedience? At least in this area he had stopped short. By the standards of his peers, he knew he could watch popular movies with racy sexual situations and still "seem" Christian. That's all he needed.

To his credit, Pete asked me what he should do. I told him to follow Mary's lead and not watch the sexy videos, and he agreed to do so.

TOGETHER ON THE MIDDLE GROUND

So often there's no challenging voice like Mary's calling us to obedience and perfection. Satisfied with mere excellence, we stop short of God's standards. We move nearer our peers only to find distance from God.

Even banded together in congregations, we stop short. Our event-driven approach in our churches feels good, but often fails to really challenge us.

My church in Des Moines has an excellent choir, known throughout our region for its professional sound. Our orchestra is even supplemented by players from the local professional symphony orchestra. In discussing our church with a new neighbor, she said, "Oh, I've been to your church. I really like it. It's just like going to a show!"

My church has an excellent schedule of tradition-driven events. There's our "Super Bowl Sunday" evening service that fosters racial harmony. We have "Honor America Night" every Fourth of July to honor our great country, inviting renowned speakers like Elizabeth Dole, Gary Bauer, and Cal Thomas. Our annual "Metro Night" honors the volunteers and staff of our daughter church in the inner city. We have Christmas specials, Easter specials, "Friends Day," "Back to School Night," and much more.

Clearly, we're striving to be "the church to belong to" in Des Moines. Have we profited? What has come from this search for excellence?

Recently, we scheduled a week of nightly all-church prayer meetings to begin the new year. Now hardly anyone would argue with the strategic value of prayer or question the fact that we're commanded as believers to be faithful at it. But obedience in the matter of prayer is costly and takes commitment. On Monday night as our week of prayer began, a mere thirty-four adults showed up out of a regular church attendance of twenty-three hundred. By Thursday, only seventeen adults were praying. I was totally discouraged. Yet one week later, on Worker Recognition Sunday, one thousand people were there to be recognized for their service in the church.

I also organized an intercessors' group during our church's Wednesday night services, simply opening a room for ninety minutes of intercession for our congregation. The first night, a half-dozen people came to the door and asked, "Is this the room where they're teaching about intercession?"

"No, we won't be *teaching* about intercession," I answered. "We're going to *be* interceding." Each person turned away to leave. It feels good to learn about intercession, but it's a costly thing to do. The same can be said about purity.

WHAT CAN WE EXPECT?

In so many areas, we're often sitting together on the middle ground of excellence, a good distance from God. When challenged by His higher standards, we're comforted that we don't look too different from those around us. Trouble is, we don't look much different from non-Christians either.

Our adolescent Christians are often indistinguishable from their non-Christian peers, sharing the same activities, music, jokes, and attitudes about premarital sex. Kristin, a teenager, told us, "Our youth group is filled with kids faking their Christian walk. They are actually taking drugs, drinking, partying, and having sex. If you want to walk purely, it's easier to hang around with the non-Christians at school than to hang around with the Christians at church. I say that because school friends know where I stand and they say, 'That's cool—I can accept that.' The Christian kids mock me, laughing and asking, 'Why be so straight? Get a life!' They pressure my values at every turn." She told us about Brad, a lay leader's son, who told her, "I know intercourse is wrong before marriage, but anything short of that is fine. I love to get up under a bra."

Sadly, the adults are no different from the Christian teens. Linda, a single career woman, says her adult singles group at church has "players"— men and women who stalk their prey to satisfy their own needs.

Christian couples have also fallen short. (*From Steve:* My daily radio talk show is filled with calls from Christians asking how they can recover from adulterous affairs or deal with a marital separation.)

Have we gone blind? What can we expect from our across-the-board commitment to the middle ground? Don't we realize that our recent converts to Christianity will become just like us? Will it be a comfort to see them just as lazy regarding their personal devotion to Jesus as we are?

And don't we realize what our slack standards are costing us in our witness to the world? In *Revival Praying,* author Leonard Ravenhill writes,

> This present day is like an arena whose terraces are filled with
> the militant godless, the brilliant and belligerent skeptics, plus
> the blank-faced heathen millions, all looking into the empty

ring to see what the Church of the living God can do. How I burn at this point! What *are* we Christians doing? To use a very tattered phrase, are we just "playing church"?

THE RIGHT RESPONSE

Israel's King Josiah was only twenty-six years of age when he faced a similar situation of neglect for God's standards. In 2 Chronicles 34 we read how a copy of God's Law—long forgotten—had been found during a large-scale renovation of the temple. Then he listened as this Law was read aloud to him—bringing inescapably to his attention God's standards and the people's failure to live up to them.

Josiah didn't say, "Oh come on, we've lived this way for years. Let's not get legalistic about all this!" No, he was horrified. He tore his robes as a sign of grief and despair. "Great is the Lord's anger," he said as he immediately acknowledged his people's negligence and sought God's further guidance.

God quickly answered with these words about Josiah's reaction:

> Because your heart was responsive and you humbled your-
> self before God when you heard what he spoke against this
> place and its people, and because you humbled yourself
> before me and tore your robes and wept in my presence, I
> have heard you, declares the LORD. (34:27)

At this point, notice how Josiah immediately led the entire nation in a thorough return to obedience to God's standards:

> Then the king…went up to the temple of the LORD with
> the men of Judah, the people of Jerusalem, the priests and
> the Levites—all the people from the least to the greatest. He

read in their hearing all the words of the Book of the Covenant, which had been found in the temple of the LORD. The king stood by his pillar and renewed the covenant in the presence of the LORD—to follow the LORD and keep his commands, regulations and decrees with all his heart and all his soul, and to obey the words of the covenant written in this book.

Then he had everyone in Jerusalem and Benjamin pledge themselves to it; the people of Jerusalem did this in accordance with the covenant of God, the God of their fathers.

Josiah removed all the detestable idols from all the territory belonging to the Israelites, and he had all who were present in Israel serve the LORD their God. As long as he lived, they did not fail to follow the LORD, the God of their fathers. (2 Chronicles 34:29-33)

No mixture there. Knowing that God's standard is the standard of true life, Josiah rose up and tore down *everything* that was in opposition to God.

COUNTING THE COST

And what about you? Now that you've heard about God's standard of sexual purity, are you willing, in the spirit of Josiah, to make a covenant to hold to that standard with all your heart and soul? Will you tear down every sexual thing that stands in opposition to God?

Can you see that you've been living the mixed standards of mere excellence? Stopping short but still looking Christian enough?

Or have you aimed for obedience and perfection, where you're truly called to go?

How will you know? By the costs you're willing to pay. What's your Christian life costing you?

It costs *something* to learn about Christ. It costs *a lot* to live like Christ.

- It costs something to join a few thousand men at a conference to sing praises to God and learn how we should live; it costs a lot to come home and remain committed to the changes you said you'd make in your life.

- It costs something to avoid *Playboy* magazine; it costs a lot to control your eyes and mind daily.

- It costs something to send your child to Christian school so others can teach your children about God; it costs a lot to have regular family devotions, complete with Dad leading worship songs and heartfelt prayer.

- It costs something to insist that your kids dress modestly; it costs a lot to make them *think* modestly and nicely.

So where do you stand? Are you comfortable? Do you have a broad tolerance of sin in your behavior? Has your approach to God led to a high level of mixture in your life?

If so, you likely have mixture in your sexual standards, and you likely have *at least a hint* of sexual impurity in your life. You won't pay the price of true obedience—like avoiding the sensuality found in many Hollywood films. Like avoiding thoughts of old girlfriends and the flirtatious woman at work. Like training your eyes to look away from string bikinis, full-busted sweaters, slick spandex, and the women who wear them.

God is your Father and expects obedience. Having given you the Holy Spirit as your power source, He believes His command should be enough for you, just as you believe your command should be enough for your kids.

Trouble is, we aren't in search of obedience. We're in search of mere excellence, and His command is *not* enough. We push back, responding, "*Why* should I eliminate every hint? That's too hard!"

We have countless churches filled with countless men encumbered by sexual sin, weakened by low-grade sexual fevers—men happy enough to go to Promise Keepers but too sickly to *be* promise keepers.

A spiritual battle for purity is going on in every heart and soul. The costs are real. Obedience is hard, requiring humility and meekness, very rare elements indeed.

We were told about James, a respected teen in his youth group, who refused to promise to stay sexually pure when pressed to do so. "There are too many unforeseen situations out there for me to make such a promise," he said. James has stopped short. Have you?

FROM FRED: WHO ARE YOU, REALLY?

Sexual impurity has become rampant in the church because we've ignored the costly work of obedience to God's standards as individuals, asking too often, "How far can I go and still be called a Christian?" We've crafted an image and may even *seem* sexually pure while permitting our eyes to play freely when no one is around, avoiding the hard work of *being* sexually pure.

From my college days, one man's example of this still serves as a warning to me. During my freshman year at Stanford, I became homesick. A dorm buddy who grew up in the shadow of the university felt sorry for me and asked me to his parents' home for dinner. They were extremely wealthy, and their home was stunning. What a great night! Not only did I have my first artichokes (which fascinate me to this day), but the mother was a strikingly pleasant host, and I learned that the father, a prominent local businessman, had a high position in their church and believed in the importance of family time.

A few weeks later, I was sitting in a barber's chair when my friend's dad walked into the shop. Being somewhat shy, I didn't say anything, and because of my wet hair and the barber's drape around my neck, he didn't recognize me. Sitting down to wait his turn, he picked up a *Playboy* magazine. I was stunned! I watched to see whether he was "just reading the articles," but he immediately turned to the centerfold, which he turned sideways to catch in its full glory.

Is this you? Is there a secret, dark side to your Christian image?

If you're a teen, are you going on missions trips during the summer but still fondling some girl's breasts in the backseat of a car?

If you're a husband, are you teaching Sunday school and being active in a men's group but fantasizing day and night about naked women?

Who are you, really?

A search for mere excellence is an inadequate approach to God, leaving us vulnerable to snare after snare. Our only hope is obedience.

If we don't kill every hint of immorality, we'll be captured by our tendency as males to draw sexual gratification and chemical highs through our eyes. (We'll discuss this in detail in the next chapter.) But we can't deal with our maleness until we first reject our right to mix standards. As we ask "How holy can I be?" we must pray and commit to a new relationship with God, fully aligned with His call to obedience.

just by being male

Even apart from our stopping short of God's standards, we find another reason for the prevalence of sexual sin among men. We got there naturally—simply by being male.

FROM FRED: OUR VERY MALENESS

Before I even knew that my wife, Brenda, was pregnant with our fourth child, I became convinced through prayer that our future child would be a boy—and our second son. I was so convinced of this that, during Brenda's pregnancy, I told this to her and to a few close friends.

As delivery day neared, the pressure rose. "Why did I tell everyone?" I whined. "What if it's a girl? What if I'm wrong?"

With the start of Brenda's labor pains, the pressure on me seemed to double every minute. Finally, standing under the bright lights of the delivery room and watching a little head crowning toward birth, I knew the moment of truth was near.

The baby came out face up. *Good,* I thought. *I'll have a perfect view.* Anxious, I gently urged Brenda, "Come on, sweetheart. Push a little more."

The shoulders emerged. *Just a few more inches,* I thought. And then? *Auugh! What are you doing, Doctor?* He turned the baby toward himself at the last moment, just as the hips and legs popped out. Now I could only see the baby's back. *C'mon, c'mon,* I cried out inside.

The doctor and nurse maddeningly said nothing. Methodically and efficiently, they dried the baby, suctioned the throat, and slapped a silly little cap on the newborn. When the doctor finally presented our new child to me, the legs were flopping apart. Immediately looking down, I just had to know.

"It's a boy!" I exclaimed.

Michael is now eight years old, and his older brother, Jasen, is sixteen, and I can assure you they definitely are both males. As I raise them, I'm aware of the natural tendencies inherent to maleness that will touch every aspect of sexual purity for them, just as they do for me.

Our very maleness—and four male tendencies in particular—represents the third reason for the pervasiveness of sexual impurity among men.

MALES ARE REBELLIOUS BY NATURE

When Paul explained to Timothy that "Adam was not the one deceived; it was the woman who was deceived and became a sinner" (1 Timothy 2:14), he was noting that Adam wasn't being tricked when he ate of the forbidden fruit in the Garden of Eden. Adam *knew* it was wrong, but he ate it anyway. In the millennia since then, all of Adam's sons tend to be just as rebellious.

Author George Gilder in *Sexual Suicide* reported that men commit more than 90 percent of major crimes of violence, 100 percent of the rapes, and 95 percent of the burglaries. Men comprise 94 percent of our drunken drivers, 70 percent of suicides, 91 percent of offenders against family and children. Most often, the chief perpetrators are single men.

Our maleness brings a natural, uniquely male form of rebelliousness. This natural tendency gives us the arrogance needed to stop short of God's standards. As men, we'll often choose sin simply because we like our own way.

MALES FIND THE "STRAIGHT" LIFE DULL AND BORING

Dr. James Dobson summed up the "straight" life well in his book *Straight Talk to Men and Their Wives:*

> The straight life for a working man…is pulling your tired frame out of bed, five days a week, fifty weeks out of the year. It is earning a two-week vacation in August, and choosing a trip that will please the kids. The straight life is spending your money wisely when you'd rather indulge in a new whatever; it is taking your son bike riding on Saturday when you want so badly to watch the baseball game; it is cleaning out the garage on your day off after working sixty hours the prior week. The straight life is coping with head colds and engine tune-ups and crab grass and income-tax forms; it is taking your family to church on Sunday when you've heard every idea the minister has to offer; it is giving a portion of your income to God's work when you already wonder how ends will meet.

To all this, most men's gut-level response is, "Get me outta here!"

While our natural rebelliousness provides the *arrogance* necessary to stop short of God's standards, our natural dislike of the straight life gives us the *desire* to stop short and to instead experience the temporary pleasures of sin. Our mixed standards provide a relief from our dulling responsibilities.

MALES HAVE A STRONG, REGULAR SEX DRIVE

In *What Wives Wish Their Husbands Knew About Women,* Dr. Dobson writes, "When sexual response is blocked, males experience an accumulating physiological pressure which demands release. Two seminal vesicles (small sacs containing semen) gradually fill to capacity; as maximum level is reached, hormonal influences sensitize the man to all sexual stimuli."

For most men, this buildup to heightened sexual desire takes only about seventy-two hours. "Many women," Dr. Dobson notes, "stand in amazement at how regularly their husbands desire sexual intercourse."

He tells a story about a young couple on a water ski trip. The husband, a neophyte on skis, thrashed about the bay for much of the afternoon as he struggled to stand. Gamely he tried and tried again, but he spent more time *in* the water than on it. The effort was obviously exhausting our sunburned hero. Meanwhile his wife turned to a friend and said, "Would you believe he'll still want it when we get home tonight?"

This pressure men experience does not justify seeking release through pornography or masturbation. The body has built-in mechanisms of release (including nocturnal emissions and overflow into the urine), and in fact I've talked with many single men who, by consistently keeping their eyes and minds pure of sensual things, haven't had sex or masturbated for years. The pressure "dries up," they say. Still, it's important for all men to realize how the cycle of pressure can escalate our sensitivity to temptation.

After having sex on Sunday night, you drive to work Monday morning and, without much reaction, notice a new billboard with a foxy babe. But after three sexless nights, seeing that babe on Thursday's drive gets your "motor" running, and she may even pop in and out of your mind all day.

"If I'm going to be out all week on business," Rob told us, "Sue and I usually have sex on Sunday night. On Monday night when I'm on the road, I have dinner, do a little work, catch CNN, and go to bed. I may think about sex, but it's not big deal. By Wednesday night, however, I'm not the same man. I practically feel possessed! The temptations are horrible, and they seem to rise in intensity each night."

Your body isn't reliable for *any* spiritual battle, much less the battle for sexual purity and obedience. We easily identify with Paul:

> When I want to do good, evil is right there with me. For in
> my inner being I delight in God's law; but I see another law
> at work in the members of my body, waging war against the
> law of my mind and making me a prisoner of the law of sin
> at work within my members. What a wretched man I am!
> (Romans 7:21-24)

Your body often breaks ranks, engaging in battle against you. This traitorous tendency pushes our sexual drive to ignore God's standards. When this sexual drive combines with our natural male arrogance and our natural male desire to drift from the straight life, we're primed and fueled for sexual captivity.

The means of ignition, meanwhile, comes from the fourth of our natural male tendencies—and the most deadly.

MALES RECEIVE SEXUAL GRATIFICATION THROUGH THE EYES

Our eyes give men the means to sin broadly and at will. We don't need a date or a mistress. We don't ever need to wait. We have our eyes and can draw sexual gratification through them at any time. We're turned on by female nudity in any way, shape, or form.

We aren't picky. It can come in a photograph of a nude stranger just as easily as in a romantic interlude with a wife. We have a visual ignition switch when it comes to viewing the female anatomy.

Women seldom understand this because they aren't sexually stimulated in the same way. Their ignitions are tied to touch and relationship. They view this visual aspect of our sexuality as shallow and dirty, even detestable. Often, any effort from husbands to put a positive spin on this "vision factor" by suggesting their wives use it to advantage in the bedroom is met with disdainful scorn. Lisa, for instance, said, "So I suppose I have to buy one of those cheap teddies and prance around like some saloon girl!"

Visual sexual gratification is no laughing matter in your fight for sexual purity. Given what the sight of nudity does to the pleasure centers of our brain, and these days it's pretty easy to see many naked or near-naked women, it's no wonder our eyes and mind resist control.

VISUAL FOREPLAY

Let's restate this fourth natural tendency in different words so you don't miss the point: *For males, impurity of the eyes is sexual foreplay.*

That's right. Just like stroking an inner thigh or rubbing a breast. Because foreplay is any sexual action that naturally takes us down the road to intercourse. Foreplay ignites passions, rocketing us by stages until we go all the way.

God views foreplay outside marriage as wrong. We get a glimpse of this in Ezekiel 23:3, where God, to portray the waywardness and apostasy of His chosen people, uses the picture of virgins in passionate sin: "In that land their breasts were fondled and their virgin bosoms caressed." (If you've ever argued that God doesn't address "petting" in the Bible, let Ezekiel 23:3 serve as a corrective to your thinking.) Just as instructive is the overall thrust of New Testament teaching on sexual purity (study again the passages listed at the end of chapter 4) and the application of their standards mentally as well as physically. From God's viewpoint, sex is more than being inside a woman.

What acts constitute foreplay? Clearly, "caressing the breasts" is foreplay. Why? Intercourse is sure to follow. If not with her tonight, then at least with masturbation later back home. If not with her tonight, then maybe tomorrow night when her will has weakened.

Masturbation while fantasizing about another woman besides your wife or "fantasy intercourse" while dreaming is the same as doing it. Remember the standard Jesus set? "You have heard that it was said, 'Do not commit adultery.' But I tell you that anyone who looks at a woman lustfully has already committed adultery with her in his heart" (Matthew 5:27-28).

What else is foreplay? Mutual stroking of the genitals is foreplay. Even stroking the top of the thigh can be foreplay. (Young men may not see it that way, but fathers do! If you saw a boy stroking your daughter's thigh, we would bet that you wouldn't just wink and turn away.) When a girl lays her head in the lap of a teenage boy, that's foreplay. A mild form, perhaps, but that'll get his motor running at levels too high for young motors. Slow dancing can be foreplay, if certain parts of the body are in close contact.

This isn't to say that young couples can't relate physically in ways that aren't foreplay, such as holding hands, walking arm in arm, or even a short kiss. But heavy kissing around the neck and chest leads naturally to stripping, which leads to mutual masturbation, which leads to intercourse.

BREAKING PROMISES

If you're married, you may be asking, What does all this have to do with me? My foreplay happens only with my wife.

Are you sure? Impurity of the eyes provides definite sexual gratification. Isn't *that* foreplay? When you see a hot movie scene, is there a twitch below your belt? What are you thinking when you're on the beach and suddenly meet a jaw-dropping beauty in a thong bikini? You gasp while Mission Control drones, "We have ignition!" You have her in bed on the spot, though only in your mind. Or you file away the image and fantasize about her later.

You stare at a sexy model and lust; you stare some more and lust some more. Your motor revs into the red zone, and you need some type of release or the engine's going to blow.

No doubt about it: Visual sexual gratification is a form of sex for men. As males, we draw sexual gratification and chemical highs through our eyes.

Alex remembers the time he was watching TV with his sister-in-law. The rest of the family was at the mall. "She was lying flat on her stomach on the floor in front of me, wearing tight shorts, and she'd fallen asleep watching TV. I was on the chair, and I happened to look down and see her upper thigh and a trace of her underwear. I tried to ignore it, but my heart started racing a little, and my eyes kept looking at the back of her upper thigh. It got so exciting that I began to stare and really lust. I had to release it somehow. I masturbated while she slept, right out in the open."

In Alex's case, impurity of the eyes was clearly foreplay, which led to further sin. It's critical to recognize visual sexual impurity as foreplay. If viewing sensual things merely provides a flutter of appreciation for a woman's beauty, it would be no different than viewing the awesome power of a thunderstorm racing over the Iowa cornfields. No sin. No problem.

But if it *is* foreplay, and if you're getting sexual gratification, it defiles the marriage bed:

> Marriage should be honored by all, and the marriage bed
> kept pure, for God will judge the adulterer and all the sexu-
> ally immoral. (Hebrews 13:4)

And it's certain you're also paying prices you may not even see:

> Do not be deceived: God cannot be mocked. A man reaps
> what he sows. The one who sows to please his sinful nature,
> from that nature will reap destruction. (Galatians 6:7-8)

Furthermore, like Alex, you're breaking promises. You promised your wife she would be your only vessel of sexual satisfaction on the face of the earth. So did Alex, but during that episode on the couch, he broke that promise. He wasn't being true to his one faithful love.

Consider this story from Ed Cole, a pastor who speaks nationally: At the close of a noon prayer meeting he'd conducted for the staff of a large ministry, a young woman drew him aside for private prayer.

"I have a problem," she told him, a little shyly.

"What's your problem?" he asked.

Her face drew tight, and tears welled up in her eyes. "I don't really know," she stammered, biting her lip, "but my husband says I have a problem."

Ed tried again. "What does your husband say your problem is?"

"He says I don't understand him," she finally said, agonizing over each word.

"What don't you understand?" Ed asked.

Suddenly the young lady began to weep bitterly, from deep within.

"My husband keeps magazines by his side of the bed," she gasped quietly between sobs. "*Playboy, Penthouse,* and those others. He says he needs to look at them before he can have sex with me. He says he needs them to stimulate him." She squeezed out the sentence, tears flowing down her face. "I told him he doesn't really need those magazines, but he says I don't understand him. He says if I really loved him, then I would understand why he has to have the magazines, and I would let him get more of them."

When Ed later inquired what her husband did for a living, she replied, "He's a youth minister."

No wife should be made to share the intimacy of her marriage bed with some shameless porn model. In this instance, the husband not only asked his wife to *accept* his sin but also to *enable* his sin by allowing him to buy more magazines. Then he justifies his behavior by blaming her. Preposterous! This man, too, was not being true to his one faithful love.

MALENESS VS. MANHOOD

If we get into sexual sin naturally—just by being male—then how do we get out? We can't eliminate our maleness, and we're sure we don't want to.

For instance, we *want* to look at our wives and desire them. They're beautiful to us, and we're sexually gratified when we gaze at them, often daydreaming about the night ahead and what bedtime will bring. In its proper place, maleness is wonderful.

Yet our maleness is a major root of sexual sin. So what do we do?

We must choose to be *more* than male. We must choose *manhood.*

When our fathers admonished us to "be a man about it," they were encouraging us to rise up to a standard of manhood they already understood. They wanted us to fulfill our potential, to rise above our natural tendencies to take the easy way out. When our fathers said, "Be a man," they were asking us to be like them.

Our heavenly Father also exhorts us to be men. He wants us to be like Him. When He calls us to "be perfect as your Father in heaven is perfect," He's asking us to rise above our natural tendencies to impure eyes, fanciful minds, and wandering hearts. His standard of purity doesn't come naturally to us. He calls us to rise up, by the power of His indwelling presence, and get the job done.

Before an important battle for the army he commanded, Joab said to the troops of Israel, "Be of good courage, and let us play the men for our people" (2 Samuel 10:12, KJV). In short, he was saying, "We know God's plan for us. Let's rise up as men, and set our hearts and minds to get it done!"

Regarding sexual integrity, God wants *you* to rise up and get it done.

choosing true manhood

You stand before an important battle. You've decided that the slavery of sexual sin isn't worth your love of sexual sin. You're committed to removing every hint of it. But how? Your maleness looms as your own worse enemy.

You got into this mess by being male; you'll get out by being a *man*.

FROM FRED: JESUS' HANDS AND EYES

What will true manhood mean, for example, in how we deal with our eyes? What are the issues?

In a newsletter, author and speaker Dr. Gary Rosberg told of seeing a pair of hands that reminded him of the hands of his father, who had gone on to heaven. Gary continued to reminisce about what his father's hands meant to him. Then he shifted his thoughts to the hands of Jesus, noting this simple truth: "They were hands that never touched a woman with dishonor."

As I read this, sorrow tore at my soul. Oh, how I wished I could say that about my hands! I have degraded women with my hands, and I regret the sin.

As I thought about it more, I realized that since my first year of salvation, I *haven't* touched a woman in dishonor. What a joy to contemplate!

I pondered Gary's words a little longer. Jesus' hands never touched a woman with dishonor, but Jesus said that lusting with the eyes is the same as touching. Given that Jesus is sinless, I suddenly realized that Jesus not only never touched a woman with dishonor, He never even *looked* at a woman in dishonor. Could I say that?

I couldn't. Though saved and free to walk purely, I had *still* chosen to look at women in dishonor.

Oh, don't be so hard on yourself, one might say. *It's natural for a male to look. That's part of our nature.* But what you're doing is *stealing.* The impure thought life is the life of a thief. You're stealing images that aren't yours. When you had premarital sex, you touched someone who didn't belong to you. When you looked down the blouse of a woman who isn't your wife, you were stealing something that isn't yours to take. It's just like walking down Main Street behind someone who drops a one-hundred-dollar bill out of his pocket, and you pick it up. That money isn't yours—*even if he didn't know he lost it.* If you choose to keep the money instead of saying, "Hey, Mister," then you've taken something you're not entitled to.

Similarly, if a woman's blouse falls open, you can't say, "Hey, that's in my sight line, I get to have that." No, you have to look away. Otherwise you're a thief. You need to leave that valuable creation in the hands of God and her husband or her future husband.

When we're thieves with our eyes, we're embezzling sexual gratification from areas that don't belong to us, from women who aren't connected to us.

In this arena, Jesus, having never looked on a woman with dishonor, is clearly our role model.

Well, sure! you say. *He was God. It's unfair to expect me to live like Him!*

Maybe. But if, because of His deity, Jesus' personal standard seems unattainable to you, let's look at another manhood role model from Scripture in the area of sexual purity.

JUST A MAN

His name was Job, and in our minds this man is the essential role model of sexual purity in Scripture. In the book of the Bible that tells his story, we see God bragging about Job to Satan:

> Have you considered my servant Job? There is no one on
> earth like him; he is blameless and upright, a man who fears
> God and shuns evil. (Job 1:8)

Was God proud of Job? You bet! He applauded His servant's faithfulness in words of highest praise. And if you walked in purity, blameless and upright, He would speak just as proudly of you. Joy would abound in His heart. You already *have* the freedom and authority to walk purely. You don't need further counseling. You don't need further deliverance.

But such a passage from Scripture may actually discourage you when you compare Job's example with your own life. So let's find out more about how Job did it.

In Job 31:1, we see Job making this startling revelation: "I made a covenant with my eyes not to look lustfully at a girl."

A covenant with his eyes! You mean he made a promise with his eyes to not gaze upon a young woman? It's not possible! It can't be true!

Yet Job was successful; otherwise, he wouldn't have made this promise:

> *"If my heart has been enticed by a woman,*
> *or if I have lurked at my neighbor's door,*
> *then may my wife grind another man's grain,*
> *and may other men sleep with her." (31:9)*

Job had been totally successful, or he could not have made this statement from his heart. He *knew* he had lived right, and he *knew* his eyes and mind were pure. He swore to it upon his wife and marriage before God and man.

Let's go back to the beginning of the story and read the opening verse of the book of Job:

> In the land of Uz there lived *a man* whose name was Job.
> This *man* was blameless and upright; he feared God and
> shunned evil.

Job was just a man! As you realize that, these precious words should gloriously flood your soul: *If he can do it, so can I.* God wants you to know that in your manhood as He created it, you, too, can rise above sexual impurity.

From Fred: Making My Covenant

When I first gave serious consideration to Job's example, I meditated upon his words for days on end. Job and I were different in only one way—our actions. God called him "blameless." I wasn't yet blameless, but I *was* a man, just as Job was, so there was hope.

After a few days, my mind turned to the word "covenant"—an agreement between God and man. *What exactly am I to do when I make a covenant?* I could say the words to make a promise, but I was uncertain whether I could keep my word.

And my eyes? Could I really expect my eyes to keep their end of the bargain? *Eyes can't think or talk! How do they keep a promise?*

Day after day, my mind returned to this covenant concept, trying to picture it, all the while remaining in my sin. Yet something was stirring deep in my soul.

I remember the moment—the exact spot on Merle Hay Road in Des Moines—when it all broke loose. I'd failed God with my eyes for the thirty-millionth time. My heart churned in guilt, pain, and sorrow. Driving down Merle Hay Road, I suddenly gripped the wheel and through clenched teeth, I yelled out: "That's it! I'm through with this! I'm making a covenant with my eyes. I don't care what it takes, and I don't care if I die trying. It stops here. It stops *here!*"

I made that covenant and built it brick by brick. Later, Steve and I will show you the blueprint for building that brick wall, but for now, study my breakthrough:

- I made a clear decision.
- I decided once and for all to make a change.

I can't describe how much I meant it. Floods of frustration from years of failure poured from my heart. I'd just had it! I wasn't fully convinced I could trust myself even then, but I'd finally and truly engaged the battle. Through my covenant with my eyes, all my mental and spiritual resources were now leveled upon a single target: my impurity.

With that covenant I had also chosen manhood, to rise above my natural male tendencies. That was a huge step for me, as you'll see later on.

THE BIBLE'S GREATEST SISSY

This step may still seem odd to you. But remember, acts of obedience will often appear strange, even illogical. We've sometimes been challenged with the words, "Who in their right mind would ever make a covenant with their eyes like this? It seems crazy."

To answer that objection, let's look at the story of the man we'll call the greatest sissy in the Bible. His name was Zedekiah, and he was reigning as king in Jerusalem at a time when the Babylonians were threatening to capture and destroy the city and bring an end to the nation of Judah.

Zedekiah's lack of manhood rose to the surface in the events described in Jeremiah 38. Jeremiah himself, as God's prophet, knew what the outcome of the Babylonian invasion would be, and he made it known:

> Jeremiah was telling all the people…"This is what the LORD
> says: 'Whoever stays in this city will die by the sword, famine
> or plague, but whoever goes over to the Babylonians will live.

He will escape with his life; he will live.' And this is what the
LORD says: 'This city will certainly be handed over to the
army of the king of Babylon, who will capture it.'" (38:1-3)

When Zedekiah heard about this, he let his officials throw Jeremiah
into a deep cistern to shut him up. He later ordered his servants to lift the
prophet out, but he still kept Jeremiah under arrest. Then one day, with
Jerusalem under siege, the king summoned Jeremiah to a secret meeting.
Jeremiah told the king what to do.

"This is what the LORD God Almighty, the God of Israel,
says: 'If you surrender to the officers of the king of Babylon,
your life will be spared and this city will not be burned
down; you and your family will live. But if you will not surrender to the officers of the king of Babylon, this city will be
handed over to the Babylonians and they will burn it down;
you yourself will not escape from their hands.'" (38:17-18)

Surrender! God, through Jeremiah, was asking the king to do something
very difficult, something that made no sense. Who in their right mind would
ever leave the fortress and go over to the enemy? It seemed crazy. Still, God's
Word was clear. The city would fall whether they stayed or left.

Zedekiah expressed his fear, but Jeremiah remained firm:

"Obey the LORD by doing what I tell you. Then it will go
well with you, and your life will be spared." (38:20)

But Zedekiah, indecisive and fearful, failed to obey. The right thing to
do was too illogical, too costly. The results for himself, his family, and his
nation were tragic.

Man's Man or God's Man?

When it comes down to it, God's definition of real manhood is pretty simple: It means hearing His Word and *doing it*. That's God's *only* definition of manhood—a doer of the Word. And God's definition of a sissy is someone who hears the Word of God and *doesn't* do it.

Have you ever known a guy whose beard is so heavy he uses two blades to shave in the morning—one for each side of his face? By late afternoon, his four o'clock shadow is so thick he has to shave again. Four blades in one day! For those of us who are "smooth men," we hold this tough guy in awe.

But God cares nothing about that. When God looks around, He's not looking for a man's man but for "God's man." His definition of a man—someone who hears His Word and acts upon it—is tough, but at least it's clear.

Meanwhile, the results of failing to be a man according to God's definition are always tragic. The fact is, as Galatians 6:7-8 tells us, God is not mocked: You *do* reap what you sow, both to the good and to the bad.

By now you understand God's command that you should eliminate every hint of sexual immorality from your life. If you do that, as Job did through his covenant with his eyes, then you're God's man. If you don't eliminate every hint, are you a sissy? Maybe so.

Earlier in the book of Jeremiah we read these desperate words spoken by the prophet to the people: "How long will you be unclean?" (13:27). That's the question for you as well: How long will you choose to be sexually unclean?

It's difficult to be victorious. We told ourselves repeatedly that we wanted out, but words are mere dandelion puffs, blowing about in the weakest breeze. Without resolute manhood girding these words, nothing happens. Talking isn't the same as doing.

In the next several chapters we'll first help you to decisively choose victory in the arena of sexual purity. Then we'll follow that up with guidelines for living out that victory as a real man.

The Heart of a Woman

As a woman, you've no doubt become aware of how much men and women differ sexually.

Heather is trying to comprehend this. "I'm starting to be more understanding and sensitive to my husband's feelings," she said. "Men are *always* in the mood."

Andrea commented, "Through the years I've come to read my husband's body signals and usually, even if I'm tired or don't feel good, I can appreciate his sexual needs, so I do my part to satisfy him. I have to admit, though, I've had times that I felt resentful, wondering why my emotional needs weren't as important as his physical needs. I've told him repeatedly what my needs are for intimacy to better satisfy him and not feel like I'm just an object for his physical pleasure. Although my husband is wonderful in so many ways, he still slips up in this area, and I have to remind him often."

Andrea warmed to the subject. "Ann Landers once ran a series of stories of women who couldn't care less about sex anymore. My husband asked me how I felt about that. I told him honestly that I could appreciate where those women are coming from sometimes. He looked surprised, but I went on to say that I could understand why they despise sex if their husbands had never done anything to please their wives, and done only what it took to satisfy themselves."

It can often be difficult for wives not to be repulsed by the male tendency to draw sexual satisfaction from the eyes.

Rhonda said, "When I first heard about how men are, it seemed so wild and unlike anything I could imagine. I had a hard time believing it and occasionally even wondered if men were making it up. But having accepted the differences, I can now say that I have a good attitude about the whole thing."

Similarly, Cathy said, "Understanding that his desires have a physiological basis has helped me be more sensitive to a very real need. I used to think that Victoria's Secret was a store for sleazy women. My husband helped me understand that my wearing 'intimate apparel' was a big plus for him. I think Christian women need to feel freer to use whatever turns their man on."

At the same time, wives have to be careful of how their appearance can turn on other men. The Bible instructs women to dress modestly (1 Timothy 2:9), but many women tend to take such verses lightly. When shopping, some women will look for "something attractive," when they really mean "something sexy." They want the sweater that sets off their breasts, the low-cut dress that sets off their hourglass figures. While these may be nice for your husband, what about the rest of the men you know?

"I don't think that most women are consciously aware of what other men are thinking," Cathy said. "Now that I know how intense the temptations are that my husband and other men face, I'm more careful how I dress."

In relation to your own husband, understanding the seventy-two-hour cycle can help you keep him satisfied. Ellen said, "His purity is extremely important to me, so I try to meet his needs so that he goes out each day with his cup full. During the earlier years, with much energy going into childcare and with my monthly cycle, it was a lot more difficult for me to do that. There weren't too many 'ideal times' when everything was just right. But that's life, and I did it anyway."

So there's a place for the quickie. While a long-term diet of drive-by sex is unhealthy, it certainly has a place in defusing the power of the seventy-two-hour temptation cycle. Sometimes you just don't have the time or energy for the full package, but if you care about his purity, you can find just enough energy to get him by.

In terms of your attire around the house, remember that his ignition is visual. You can get his motor running just changing shirts in his presence. As Ellen said, "For my husband's sake, I try not to undress in front of him unless I'm ready for action!"

When you want your husband to watch romantic videos with you, be especially sensitive to how movies with vivid love scenes will subject him to visual sensuality. Of course you want the two of you to watch the movie together, but give him room to say no for the sake of his sexual integrity.

Finally, as you struggle with your emotions to fully understand your husband's "problem" and its effects on your marriage, realize that something just as harmful to marriage as sexual sin is the sin of comparison. When men look at sensual things, it can make them less satisfied with their wives. Likewise when women fantasize about the perfect husband, it can make them less satisfied with the mate God has given them.

Women are susceptible to this in different ways. Some fall prey to comparing their now-stodgy husband to the "hunk" they once knew in college. For others, the dissatisfaction comes from dreaming of a fling to a far-off island, or reading a romance novel and responding with "if only" feelings that lead only to dissatisfaction.

Andrea agreed that, for her, a big potential downfall "would be fantasizing about the 'perfect husband,' especially during trying times in our marriage. This makes me feel dissatisfied with him, and I want more from him than I should."

Frances admitted that women can "fall short in our thought lives. We compare our husbands with other women's husbands, but not necessarily in the physical or sexual arenas. We do it spiritually, comparing whose husband is a better spiritual leader, or just more spiritual in general. We also compare our lives with other women's lives—like who has it easier, and who does and doesn't have to work outside the home. That also can cause dissatisfaction with our husbands."

PART III

choosing victory

the time to decide

We came across a newspaper story about a World War II vet named B. J. "Bernie" Baker who was told he was dying of bone cancer. Given only two years to live, he told the doctors to fight the disease with everything possible. "Give me the treatments," he said. "I'll keep living my life." Meanwhile he and his wife found time for a motor-home drive to Alaska, a fishing excursion to Costa Rica, and several trips to Florida.

Nine years after the diagnosis, he was struggling with shortage of breath and loss of strength but said, "I'm going to keep fighting. Might as well."

Those words were not said in resignation. They were the words of a fighter, a real man, a man who had faced bombs and machine-gun fire in the South Pacific before returning to America and eventually starting Baker Mechanical Company with two pipe wrenches and a $125 pickup truck. (It would become one of the largest companies of its kind in America.) The cancer hit him hard, but he had no plans for surrender.

Might as well keep fighting. What was B. J.'s alternative?

To quit and die.

What about you, in your battle with impure eyes and mind? What's your alternative to fighting?

To stay ensnared and die spiritually.

When you talk to courageous men from B. J.'s generation, World War II veterans who embody the title of Tom Brokaw's book *The Greatest*

Generation, they say they don't feel like heroes. They simply had a job to do. When the landing-craft ramps fell open, they swallowed hard and said, "It's time." Time to fight.

In your struggle with sexual impurity, isn't it time? Sure, fighting back will be hard. It was for us. When we began our fight, we fully expected to take a beating at first, and we did. Our sin had humbled us. But we wanted victory over that sin and the respect of our God.

Your life and home are under a withering barrage of machine-gun sexuality that rakes the landscape mercilessly. Right now you're in a landing craft, inching closer to shore and a showdown. God has given you the weapons and trained you for battle.

You can't stay in the landing craft forever. Sooner or later, the ramp will drop, and then it will be your time to run bravely into the teeth of battle. God will run *with* you, but He won't run *for* you.

It's time to plunge ahead and go like a man.

From Fred: Winning When the Battle Is Hottest

If you remember my story, I rejected *some* sexual sin when I became a Christian. But I hadn't *entirely* destroyed my yielding to our sexual culture's negative influence upon me, and so I became ensnared. As I continued to fight sexual temptation as a married man, many a day I wistfully mourned, *A hormone drop would really help.* I was tired of the battle and wanted it badly to go away.

Eventually, as the birthdays passed and nothing cleared up, I sensed I'd been duped. I was sick of sinning, sick of Satan, and sick of me, and I didn't want to wait anymore. Like the people of Israel, I came to loathe myself. (Just like the people of Israel, according to God's prophecy in Ezekiel 6:9.)

I was angry. I wanted to win right away and to win decisively—not somewhere down the road where age might bring victory through the back door. I wanted to win when the battle was hottest.

You should too. If you don't win now, you'll never know whether you're truly a man of God.

Going to War, Going to Win

Three years ago I counseled Ben, who said he wanted sexual integrity, but his words were just words. "I'm still buying the *Playboy*s," he said recently. "I guess I just don't hate them enough."

Kirk, a worker in a local ministry, was caught in the early stages of an affair. By talking dirty, he'd been pushing a coworker toward a compromising situation. He said he wanted my help, and I agreed to meet with Kirk and his pastor.

In our first meeting the pastor said, "In our community, this kind of talk and behavior is commonplace." I saw Kirk nod his head in agreement. I didn't meet with Kirk again because I knew he didn't hate his sin.

Similarly, I'm reminded of seventeen-year-old Ronnie, who was masturbating several times a day. His pastor told me, "Ronnie *says* he wants to be free, but he doesn't feel any compunction to put in any effort on his own. He'll give up his sin, but only if God does it." Later, Ronnie rushed into his pastor's office in terror, saying, "Pastor, you've got to help me! You know the fantasies I have while masturbating? Two weeks ago, they suddenly turned homosexual, and I can't make them stop!" That was the epiphany that Ronnie needed to stand up and fight.

We've known those who have failed in their battle for sexual purity, and we know some who have won. The difference? Those who won hated their impurity. They were going to war and were going to win—or die trying. Every resource was leveled upon the foe.

There will be no victory in this area of your life until you choose manhood with all your might.

WHY NOT NOW?

Leading up to a decisive choice for sexual purity, we must make some hard choices and answer some hard questions:

- How long do I intend to stay ensnared?
- How long must my family wait?
- How long before I can look God in the eye?

My wife, Brenda, asked me one of those hard questions a few years ago. Although it was focused on something other than sexual sin, the story behind it illustrates the hard decisions necessary to escape sexual bondage.

When I reached age thirty-five, the lack of my father's acceptance suddenly rocked me deeply. This pain affected my relationship with my wife and kids. I was harsh in my tone, harsh in my words. Harsh, harsh, harsh. Brenda tried to explain away my behavior, but after a year she became frustrated. One day she told me, "All right, then! Fine. Just tell all of us how long you plan to stay like this, so we can prepare for it!" Then she stormed out of the room.

I sat there speechless for quite some time. How long *was* I going to stay like this? Ten years? Why ten? Why not five? If I could decide to change at the end of five years, why not after one? And if after one, why not now?

After her single stiletto question to my heart, I knew it was time. Starting immediately, I found a counselor. Shortly afterward I attended a Promise Keepers conference in Boulder, Colorado. That first night God spoke to me through the speaker and revealed an aspect of His love for me that I'd never understood. Sitting that evening in the bleachers at the University of Colorado's Folsom Field, the pain from my dad began dispersing. My family deserved more. I had to act decisively.

MORE QUESTIONS

Similarly, in the arena of sexual purity, you're at your own point of decision.

Admit it: You love your sexual highs, but slavery engulfs you. Is the love worth the loathing? Is stopping short of God's standards right?

Look in the mirror. Are you proud of your sexual fantasizing? Or do you feel degraded after viewing lingerie ads or sex scenes in films?

Sexually speaking, you have a low-grade sexual fever. It doesn't disable you, but you aren't healthy either. You can sort of function normally, but you can't really push hard. Basically, you just get by. And if this fever doesn't break, you'll never fully function as a Christian. Like the prodigal, you need to come to your senses and make a decision.

Your own wife may not be aware of your problem with sexual impurity, so we'll ask the questions for her:

- How long are you going to stay sexually impure?
- How long will you rob your wife sexually?
- How long will you stunt the growth of oneness with your wife, a oneness you promised her years ago?

God's view is simple here. You need to face those questions and make a decision. Yet you're hesitating. We know you are, because we hesitated for years. You're thinking, *Wait a minute. I'm not ready.* Or, *It just isn't that easy!*

Fine. We'll agree that choosing to stop sinning doesn't always seem like a small decision. Once you're ensnared, everything looks complex. But listen to the following words spoken by preacher Steve Hill, who was addressing escape from addiction to drugs and alcohol as well as from sexual sin:

> There's no temptation that is uncommon to man. God will send you a way of escape, but you've got to be willing to take that way of escape, friend....
>
> I was an alcoholic to the max. I would drink whiskey,

straight whiskey, every day. And I was a junkie. Cocaine up my nose, in my arm, I did it all, friend. And God never delivered me from the desire and the love of drugs. He never did. What happened is that I *decided* to never touch the stuff or drink booze again....

Those of you that are into pornography may be asking God to take away your lustful desires. You are a man with hormones. You *feel* things. You have since you were a teenager, and you will until the day you die! You are attracted to the opposite sex.

I'm not saying that God cannot take the desire from you. He can! He's just never done it in my life or the tens of thousands of people I've worked with over the years. That includes pornographers. Ninety-nine percent of them had to *make a decision.* They had to make a decision to not walk by magazine racks of adult magazines and to stay faithful to their wives and their family.

We agree. It's time to make a decision. When will *you* change? How long will you wait? Five years? One year? Why not now?

THIS IS YOUR MOMENT

Consider the example of Eleazar, one of David's "three mighty men," in this brief record of a tough battle against the Philistines:

> Then the men of Israel retreated, but he stood his ground and struck down the Philistines till his hand grew tired and froze to the sword. The LORD brought about a great victory that day. (2 Samuel 23:9-10)

Eleazar refused to be ensnared anymore. Everyone else was running from the enemy, but he put his foot down and said, "I've had it with this running. I'm going to fight until I drop dead or until I drop to the field in victorious exhaustion. This is my moment to live or die."

Have you had it with the running? Author and pastor Jack Hayford once sat in his car after a banking transaction with a lovely bank teller and said to himself, "I'm either going to have to purify my mind and consecrate myself unto God, or I'm going to have to masturbate right here." That Jack could say this in front of tens of thousands of men at a Promise Keepers conference was inspirational.

How about you? How long will you allow the Philistines to chase you? Are you motivated instead to fight?

FROM FRED: MOTIVATED TO WIN

Here's a story of someone who became *very* motivated to change. Several weeks prior to his planned wedding, Barry heard me give a talk on sexual purity. My words weighed heavily on his heart because he was having a problem with R-rated movies. He had been planning to marry Heather with his secret safely tucked away, but now he decided to tell her the truth. Heather recalls her reaction to Barry's confession: "I was shocked and numb when we talked in the car that night. I just stared straight ahead, no feelings at all. After dropping him off, I cried and cried, refusing to talk to him for days. When I did agree to see him, he commented to me that I looked pretty. I got so mad and repulsed by him that I threw the engagement ring in his face and told him to get out of my sight. I felt sick and dirty."

As you can see, this topic is an emotional one. Women take it *personally* when they find out what men are doing in secret.

Heather asked Brenda and me to meet with her, which we did. After much prayer and counseling, Heather gave Barry a deadline of one week.

Then I met with Barry. "Can you help me?" he asked. "I'm absolutely hooked on sexy movies. I expected Heather to understand, but she was horrified and called me a pervert. Fred, I'm desperate! The invitations have already been sent out, but if I don't get this stopped, I'll have to somehow explain all this to my mother-in-law! You've got to help me!"

Do you suppose Barry was motivated? He surely was. Rarely have I met with someone who wanted to win a war more quickly. And he defeated his problem. He became a man of sexual integrity, and today he and Heather have a wonderful marriage.

You can win the war as well—and start winning it now.

ALL YOU NEED

As the basis for your victory, did you know that God has provided you with everything you need for a life of purity? And it's better than a state-of-the-art GPS navigational system.

At Calvary, He purchased for you the freedom and authority to live in purity. That freedom and that authority are His gift to you through the presence of His Spirit, who took up residence within you when you gave your life to Christ. The freedom and authority are wrapped up in our new inner connection to His divine nature, which is the link that gives us His power and the fulfillment of His promises:

> His divine power has given us everything we need for life
> and godliness through our knowledge of him who called us
> by his own glory and goodness. Through these he has
> given us his very great and precious promises, so that
> through them you may participate in the divine nature and
> escape the corruption in the world caused by evil desires.
> (2 Peter 1:3-4)

It's like the situation facing Joshua and the people of Israel as they prepared to cross the Jordan River and possess the Promised Land. What did God say to Joshua?

> Have I not commanded you? Be strong and courageous!
> Do not be terrified; do not be discouraged, *for the* LORD
> *your God will be with you wherever you go.* (Joshua 1:9)

He'd given the Israelites all they needed. They merely had to cross the river.

Regarding sexual purity, God knows the provision He's made for us. We aren't short on power or authority, but what we lack is *urgency.* We must choose to be strong and courageous to walk into purity. In the millisecond it takes to make that choice, the Holy Spirit will start guiding you and walking through the struggle with you.

GOD IS WAITING

Each one of us has been manipulated by our sexual culture; each of us has made choices to sin. To varying degrees, each of us became ensnared by these choices, but we can overcome this affliction. Far too often, however, we ignore our own responsibility in this. We complain, "Well, *of course* I want to be free from impurity! I've been to the altar 433 times about it, haven't I? It just doesn't seem to be God's will to free me."

Not God's will? That's an offense to the character of God. Don't blame God.

God's will is for you to have sexual purity, though you may not think so since this hasn't been your constant experience. But He *has* made a provision for that purity. Listen to these scriptures:

> Count yourselves dead to sin but alive to God in Christ
> Jesus. Therefore do not let sin reign in your mortal body so

that you obey its evil desires. Do not offer the parts of your body to sin, as instruments of wickedness, but rather offer yourselves to God, as those who have been brought from death to life; and offer the parts of your body to him as instruments of righteousness. For sin shall not be your master, because you are not under law, but under grace. (Romans 6:11-14)

You have been set free from sin and have become slaves to righteousness. (Romans 6:18)

God is waiting for you. But He is not waiting by the altar, hoping you'll drop by and talk for a while. He is waiting for you to rise up and engage in the battle. We have power through the Lord to overcome every level of sexual immorality, but if we don't utilize that power, we'll never break free of the habit.

You see, sexual impurity isn't like a tumor growing out of control inside us. We treat it that way when our prayers focus on *deliverance,* as we plead for someone to come remove it. Actually, sexual impurity is a series of bad decisions on our part—a result of immature character—and deliverance won't deliver you into instant maturity. Character work needs to be done.

How do you do that character work? That's what we'll explore in the rest of this book.

Holiness is not some nebulous thing. It's a series of right choices. You needn't wait for some holy cloud to form around you. You'll be holy when you choose not to sin. You're already free from the *power* of sexual immorality; you are not yet free from the *habit* of sexual immorality, until you choose to be—until you say, "That's enough! I'm choosing to live purely!"

regaining what was lost

Okay, so you've decided it's time to fight. And you realize that your battle for sexual purity will cost you something. It will require sacrifice, intensity, and honor.

But let's get something else in clear view: What can you expect to *gain* by choosing manhood and the purity that goes with it?

By winning this war, your life will be blessed in tremendous ways. Your victory will recover what was lost through sin. Victory will help you…

- regain and revitalize your relationship with God
- regain and revitalize your relationship with your wife
- regain and revitalize your relationship with your children
- regain and revitalize your relationship to your ministry

FROM FRED: NEW LIGHT AND LIGHTNESS

Because of sin, I hadn't been able to look at myself in a mirror for years. While I knew God loved me unconditionally, I also knew He didn't unconditionally approve of my behavior. Consequently, I couldn't look God in the eye.

Once I heard a pastor preach, "When Jesus knocks, He wants freedom to enter every room in your house. In every part of your life, He wants to be welcome and comfortable. Is He locked out of any room in your house?"

Yes, I thought to myself in the pew. *The sex chamber. It's locked tight.* I'd kept that room private, since I was a fake and a hypocrite. In one sense that didn't matter with God; I knew He loved me no matter what. But I also knew my sin caused my relationship with Him to suffer. When my own children disobey, our relationship suffers. Afterward, they look into my eyes in search of forgiveness and a restoration of our relationship. I knew I needed to do that with God.

In my situation, however, I no longer had the courage to look into His eyes for forgiveness. I was too embarrassed, having repeatedly apologized to Him but never changing. In my mind, I heard His haunting words: *Why do you call me "Lord, Lord," and do not do what I say?*

I was a prodigal eating old cobs of corn left in a pigsty. To restore my relationship with my Father, I had to get up out of the mud and start walking home. I didn't have to clean myself up first, but I did have to make that first step. On the road ahead, the Father would be waiting with a ring, a robe, shoes, and everything else an honored son was meant to have. But first I had to come to my senses, as I did that day on Merle Hay Road when I took my first step toward home—toward purity—by making that covenant with my eyes.

Before long I felt a new light and lightness in my soul. My sexual sin had brought a darkness so deep and smothering that when it vanished, the difference was so real I could practically touch it. I felt loved *and* approved by God.

Along with inner peace comes an outer peace that affects your daily life. In an earlier chapter I mentioned a businessman named Wally and his dread of hotels. Wally can now check into a hotel at night, enjoy a meal at the coffee shop, go back to his room, shower, turn out the lights, and fall asleep. "I no longer fear hotel rooms in the slightest," he says. "Sensual things don't dominate my day as they once could. All those compelling desires that ruled me are gone, and yet my desire for my wife, Tina, still percolates rather nicely!"

You'll see the same positive impact on your desire for your wife with your victory in sexual purity.

MY CAPTIVATING WIFE

Early in my marriage, I never fully gave myself emotionally to Brenda. I once thought this was the result of some personality quirk of mine, but as it turns out, it was my sexual sin that held me back. Trust now comes more naturally since I've fully released myself to Brenda and forsaken my rights to a "private" sex life with my eyes and mind.

Another reward is that Brenda no longer has fears about my having affairs with other women. Since we've talked so much and so openly about my commitment to purity, her heart is at total ease. I don't get caught up in admiring the beauty of other women, and I don't talk about other women. Since I've starved my eyes of everything sensual (except for her), I find her absolutely captivating, and she knows it.

FROM STEVE: FULL CONNECTION

I experienced a similar story. One of the things I brought into my marriage with Sandy was a secret compartment I'd guarded for years. Inside it was a girlfriend from much earlier in my life, the first true love I really had. I didn't fantasize about her, but I considered this secret compartment to be mine forever, a private place out of which I could draw fond old memories of what life was like with her.

It wasn't until I was willing to give up that secret compartment that I was fully able to connect with Sandy. Once that happened, I no longer wanted to contact my old girlfriend because I was focused on Sandy and wanting her.

Perhaps you also have secret compartments labeled Old Girlfriends or Pornography or Favorite Web Sites. You must forsake these private, secret compartments, because they're harmful.

FRIENDS WHO TRUST

Your sexual purity will also mean regaining your relationship to your friends.

Both Fred and I know that if a friend ever had to leave one of us alone in a hotel room with his wife for an evening, he could be fully assured that nothing dishonorable would happen. That was not always the case. Of course, that scenario will never happen, but that's not the point. We simply know that we're trustworthy now. Our friends don't have to worry about us "undressing their wives" in our minds or daydreaming of what it might be like to be making love to one of them.

Trust is important in the body of Christ. In 1 Corinthians 6:15-20, Paul says that not only does a sexually immoral man sin against his own body, but he also sins against the body of Christ and his friends within the body.

Our friends trust us to be pure; a failure would crush their spirits as well as our own. We must be trustworthy.

FROM FRED: YOUR LEGACY

In your relationships with your children, the knowledge that you could break patterns of generational sin is wondrous. Consider what the psalmist wrote:

As for man, his days are like grass...
    But from everlasting to everlasting
the LORD'*s love is with those who fear him,*
    and his righteousness with their children's children.
    (Psalm 103:15,17)

God is obviously interested in saving you as an individual. After all, He sent His son to die for you—personally. But He's equally interested in you as a link in an important chain because God knows that a Christian legacy, when passed on, has the power to change generations for the good.

Likewise, sin can affect families for generations, as it did in mine. I came from a family in which the men loved sex and pornography and ditched their wives or were caught up in affairs.

Having followed in their footsteps, I can still remember the pictures I viewed in *Playboy* and *Gallery* magazines more than twenty years ago. I can also remember the many girlfriends and our moments in bed. But the Lord and I won, and the generational sin was broken.

My sixteen-year-old son, Jasen, is now a handsome, strapping, six-foot adolescent with an easy smile and friendly ways. Not long ago Jasen was with friends who had some pornography. He walked away. *My son walked away.* You don't understand what that means to me!

If you're coming out of generational sin, you must continue to fight the good fight—for your children and for your children's children.

A man once said to D. L. Moody, "The world has not yet seen what God can do with a man fully devoted to Him." Moody responded, "I am that man!" Unlike Moody, young men today are spending so much of their spiritual energy fighting off sexual fevers. What if your son were kept free from this draining fever in the first place, and all of his spiritual energy could be spent on God's call in His kingdom?

It can be done. The world has not yet seen what God can do with an army of young men free of sexual fevers. If you're a father, have you worked hard enough to keep your son pure so that he might qualify for such an army? Can you yourself answer as Moody did, "I am that man"?

A Share in Building the Kingdom

After my salvation, I had a deep excitement for Christ and thought about entering full-time ministry. I looked into schools and seminaries, excited at the thought of spending my time telling everyone about Christ Jesus. Having been freed from a ruggedly promiscuous lifestyle, I found God's forgiveness to be intoxicating.

But then I was brought back to earth as I read in Scripture a conversation King David had with his son, Solomon. David is recounting what God had told him years earlier, through the prophet Nathan, regarding David's desire to build the Jewish temple:

> David said to Solomon: "My son, I had it in my heart to
> build a house for the Name of the LORD my God. But
> this word of the LORD came to me: 'You have shed much
> blood and have fought many wars. You are not to build a
> house for my Name, because you have shed much blood
> on the earth in my sight.'" (1 Chronicles 22:7-8)

Because David was a man of war and had shed much blood, he was not to build the temple. That task, God told David, was reserved for his son Solomon:

> "But you will have a son who will be a man of peace and
> rest, and I will give him rest from all his enemies on every

side.… He is the one who will build a house for my
Name." (1 Chronicles 22:9-10)

I wasn't spoken to directly by a prophet as David was, but this verse jumped off the page to me. It seemed clear that God was telling me something like this:

David was a man of war and had shed much blood, so I
could not have him build my temple. Similarly, you are a
man of deep sexual sin. I cannot have you, at this time,
building my kingdom full time. I want you to first learn to
be a simple pillar in a local church. If you are faithful, your
son will help build my kingdom full time.

This was devastating to me, but I was certain I'd heard Him correctly. Fortunately, David's great heart inspired me.

As I meditated on these verses, I decided to joyfully do the next best thing. Since I couldn't work full time building the kingdom, I could prepare my son Jasen as best I could. I set my heart diligently as David did with Solomon, helping Jasen with Bible reading, memory work, music lessons, and church attendance. I invited missionaries to stay in our home so Jasen could hear how they were impacting people's lives. Most of all, I did my best to keep him pure. I watched whom he played with, explained the dangers of pornography, and kept him from viewing sensual films and television shows.

I have to be a good example because I remember how it was with Dad and me. Early in life, Dad promised me one hundred dollars upon graduation from high school if I never smoked or drank. I never did smoke or drink through high school, and on graduation day he paid up. But what happened in college? I never started smoking, but I did start drinking. Why did I start one and not the other?

When I was ten years old, I watched Dad, a two-pack-a-day smoker, receive the news that he had six months to live. Doctors removed a lung, and I watched him endure pain resulting from the operation. Dad, who had failed several attempts to stop smoking, suddenly quit cold turkey. He never smoked again. While the particular lung disease he contracted wasn't directly caused by smoking, the dangers of smoking and my father's heroic effort to survive made a deep impression on me.

What about alcohol? Dad told me I shouldn't drink, but when he mowed the lawn or went fishing, he always capped the day with a beer or two. From my earliest age, whenever we went to restaurants, Dad ordered a martini. The unique shape of the glass, the olive, and the whole aura—shaken but not stirred—was glamorous to my young mind.

When my time of decision came with alcohol, I couldn't think of a single person who didn't drink. Certainly not my dad. No example in my life spoke about *not* drinking, so I started.

When your son questions what he should watch, what he should do with the pornography other boys show him, or what he should do when that cute girl gets him alone and starts unbuttoning her blouse, will anyone be speaking against it? It won't be his friends. Even his *church* buddies will tell him to go for it. *Your* voice had better be loud and crystal clear because it will probably be the only one whispering, "Flee immorality, son." Your *example* must be the argument opposing temptation.

AVOIDING THE CARNAGE

I'm working diligently to prepare Jasen for work in God's kingdom, knowing that for the time being I myself won't be having any broad leadership in ministry.

There were times, I must admit, that I didn't understand why this was true. But I came to a better understanding when I saw the fall of other prominent Christian leaders, when I witnessed the divorce of two key couples involved in marriage ministry at my church, and when two of my own pastors fell to adultery as well. One of them was our senior pastor, and it took our church more than a decade to fully recover. The other was an associate pastor; I saw the results of his sin up close since I was part of a recovery team to help restore him to the ministry. I remember thinking how, until that time, I'd never truly understood the word "carnage."

While I once chafed under God's limits for me in ministry, I don't chafe anymore. I know that as a premarriage teacher at my church, where I instruct thirty couples a year, any personal fall into sin would have ramifications rippling across the church. And I've known since the beginning that as I teach on purity in my church, I'd better be strong.

It's Time

God is waiting to bless you.

Your wife needs you to step up.

Your kids need you to break generational sin.

Your church needs you to serve.

Do you agree it's time?

Good. Let's put together a battle plan. The landing-craft ramps are falling open, and it's time to hit the beach.

your battle plan

Before we started winning our own battles for purity, we had a number of false starts—partly because we hadn't really made a decision. We sort of wanted purity, and sort of didn't. We didn't understand the enemy and how to approach it. The whole business of sexual integrity was mysterious.

Let's say you're in the landing craft ready to attack your sexual sin. You've made your decision. You've decided to follow your leaders as you storm the beach. The landing-craft ramp falls open. With a shout, you step courageously into the fray. But, unknown to you, the deceptive ocean currents have flushed a deep hole on the ocean floor right in front of the landing craft. You have no idea what's happened, but you're suddenly in water over your head, and the weight of your pack is sending you to the bottom. You're drowning.

Your battle is over before you even took a second step.

Satan's greatest weapon against you is just such deception. He knows Jesus has already purchased your freedom. He also knows that once you see the simplicity of this battle, you'll win in short order, so he deceives and confuses. He tricks you into thinking you're a helpless victim, someone who'll need years of group therapy. He tells you that sexual sin is just part of being a man, and there's nothing you can do about it. He tells you all about sexual addiction and makes you believe that you're not a sex addict, that you're off the hook, that you don't need an obedient life. And such deception is only one of the ways that he tries to beat you.

This chapter will remove the mystery surrounding the enemy as you launch into battle. We'll define your actual objective in practical terms, and we'll describe some critical attributes of your sexual sin. Pay close attention to these details, because once you step into the fray, you want to come out of this victorious.

YOUR OBJECTIVE IN THIS WAR

Your goal is sexual purity. Here's a good working definition of it—good because of its simplicity: *You are sexually pure when no sexual gratification comes from anyone or anything but your wife.*

Purity means stopping sexual gratification that comes to us from outside our marriage. But how to do we stop it?

We're able to draw outside sexual gratification from only two places: the *eyes* and the *mind.* Therefore, to be successful in the battle for our sexual perimeter, we must blockade the "shipping lanes" of the eyes and mind. Beyond that, we also want to make sure that we have healthy, positive affections and attitudes in our relationships with our wives. In other words, we want our *hearts* to be right.

That means your objective in the war against lust is *to build three perimeters of defense* into your life:

1. With your eyes.
2. In your mind.
3. In your heart.

Think of the first perimeter (your eyes) as your outermost defense, a wall with "Keep Out" signs around it. It defends your eyes by covenant (as Job did: "I made a covenant with my eyes not to look lustfully at a girl"), and you do that by training your eyes to *bounce* from objects of lust. Your eyes must bounce from the sensual, something they aren't currently doing. We'll explain this thoroughly in part 4.

With the second perimeter (your mind), you don't so much block out the objects of lust, but you *evaluate* and *capture* them. A key verse to support you here is 2 Corinthians 10:5: "We take captive every thought to make it obedient to Christ." You must train your mind to take thoughts captive, something it doesn't currently do. You'll learn much more about this in part 5.

Your third objective (which we'll investigate in part 6) is to build your innermost defense perimeter—in your heart. This perimeter is built by strengthening your affections for your wife and your commitment to the promises and debts you owe her. Your marriage can die from within if you neglect your promise to love, honor, and cherish your wife. *Honoring* and *cherishing* are your key actions in establishing this defense perimeter. (And this applies even if you're single: You want to honor and cherish every date, just as you hope every guy is honoring and cherishing *your* future wife when he goes out with her.)

So there's your battle plan. That's it. Nothing more, nothing less. Setting up defense perimeters and choosing not to sin. You'll have freedom from sexual impurity as soon as those defense perimeters are in place. Sexually, your *outer* life will finally match the *inner* life God created in you.

Because of your long struggle with sexual impurity, this attack plan may seem too simple to be effective. No matter. As you study the attributes of your enemy, you'll realize that simplicity is more than sufficient.

So before we move on to how to build the three defense perimeters, let's remove the mystery surrounding sexual sin by gaining a better understanding of the enemy, that we might not be deceived.

IMPURITY IS A HABIT

Some may think that impurity is genetic, like the color of our eyes. *I'm male, so I'll have impure eyes and an impure mind.* But we can't blame our roving eyes on genetics, even though men are definitely more visually oriented than women. Some men see themselves as victims of impure eyes and thoughts, as if that excuse absolved them from all responsibility.

The simple truth? Impurity is a habit. It *lives* like a habit. When some hot-looking babe walks in, your eyes have the bad habit of bouncing toward her, sliding up and down. When some glistening jogger runs past you, your eyes habitually run away with her. When the *Sports Illustrated* swimsuit issue arrives in your mailbox, out of habit you fantasize over the curves and crevices, fondling every glossy image.

The fact that impurity is merely a habit comes as a surprise to many men. It's like discovering that the big bully has a glass chin and that you don't have to cower anymore.

If impurity were genetic or some victimizing spell, you'd be helpless. But since impurity is a habit, it can be changed. You have hope, because if it *lives* like a habit, it can *die* like a habit. (We believe it can be done in six weeks.)

This is great news since habit-breaking is familiar ground, hardly mysterious. We've all dealt with bad habits. What do you do with them? You simply replace them with new and better ones. That's it. If you can practice this new habit with great focus for a month to six weeks, soon the old habit will seem unnatural.

Sexual impurity is not a "sickness" or "imbalance" for most men. Our eyes love the sexual, and our bad habits arise from our maleness. We have the bad habit of seeking cheap thrills from any dark corner we stumble into. We've habitually chosen the wrong way, and now we must habitually choose the right way.

Don't misunderstand. We're not saying your habits have no relationship to your emotions or circumstances. Glen told us, "My sexual sin became much worse when I was under a deadline at work, and especially when my wife and I fought or I felt unloved and unappreciated. It seemed at those times that I was compelled to sin sexually and couldn't say no. Honestly, I didn't think that would ever change simply by changing the habits of my eyes. But guess what? Once I got my eyes under control, these same deadlines and fights no longer compelled me sexually. My impurity just seemed to wither away on its own."

For Glen, job-related stress and lack of acceptance were not the *root* cause of his sexual impurity. The sexual impurity was simply one way he dealt with these emotions and circumstances. In short, he ran to impurity as an escape. But when he removed the sexual impurity, he began processing these things in other ways.

WORKING LIKE A HABIT

Impurity not only lives like a habit, it also *works* like a habit. The same is also true for *purity;* it *works* like a habit.

What do we mean?

Once we set a habit in concrete, we can forget about it. The habit will take care of business with little conscious thought, enabling us to focus our attention on other things. For example, we all have a habitual way of getting up in the morning. Many of us slowly climb out of bed, brush our teeth, take a shower, get dressed, and eat Wheaties with the kids at 7:10 A.M. We don't even have to think about it. We could do our morning routine in our sleep, and we usually do!

While sexual impurity works like a *bad* habit, sexual *purity* works like a *good* habit.

This should be encouraging to you. As you enter the fight against impurity, the exhausting battle might have you saying to yourself, "I can't work this hard at purity the rest of my life." But if you can just hang in there a little longer, the habit of purity will get a foothold and fight *for* you, requiring much less conscious effort.

Currently, your impure habits claw and clutch; you sin without even thinking. For instance, your eyes bounce to any short skirt that moseys by. Without thinking, your bad habits start kicking in. But with the habit of purity in place, when a woman's dress flies up on a windy day, you'll look away automatically without even thinking. If you wanted to peek, you'd have to *force* your eyes to do so.

FROM FRED: FORCING A LOOK

Hard to imagine? Then consider this little story.

After training my eyes to look away, I was sunbathing with Brenda on a Florida beach. Brenda called my attention to a bikini-clad woman approaching us. "Fred, look! You won't believe this!"

I turned to look, but initially I couldn't. The good habits had become so strong I had to force my eyes to look.

"She's way too old to wear that!" Brenda said about the sixty-something woman. I'm not sure what surprised me more: having to force my eyes to look at a woman in a bikini or seeing someone that old wearing something that skimpy.

IMPURITY FIGHTS LIKE AN ADDICTION

Impurity of the eyes and mind lives like a habit but *fights* like an addiction. Many habits are addictive. Smokers get the urge to smoke. Drug users "get a jones." Alcoholics get the shakes.

For overcoming some addictions, the addictive source can be gradually reduced. For others, the best method is cold turkey. What works best with sexual impurity? Cold turkey. You cannot just taper down. We tried. It didn't work, because we found our minds and eyes were too tricky and deceitful. With tapering, whatever impurity you *do* allow seems to multiply in its impact, and the habit won't break. Besides, tapering down also brings with it the possibility of sexual binges that might go on for days.

Binges crush your spirit. "I used to try to stop my sexual sin without really understanding what I was fighting," said Cliff. "I might grit my teeth and do well for a while, but then suddenly, maybe because I hadn't had sex in a while or because of some lustful thoughts that just got carried away, I would masturbate. Then I would say to myself, 'Well, since I failed, I might as well fail big.' I would masturbate two, three times a day for the next week or two before I could get back the strength to fight again. I can't tell you how many times I've binged like this."

Cold turkey it must be. But how? By totally starving your eyes of all things sensual besides your wife. For singles, this means starving your eyes of all things sensual. This will help you overcome the desire for premarital sex with the women you date. If you starve your eyes just like the married guys, you'll see your date as a person and not an object.

We'll teach you how to starve your eyes in part 4, but for now, know that you can expect an inner "urge to fail." You're accustomed to satisfying a portion of your sexual hunger through your eyes, anytime and anywhere you please. Your body will fight for these highs. As you advance in purity, that part of your sexual hunger, once fed by your eyes, remains unfed and doesn't just disappear. This demanding hunger runs to the only available pantry left to you: your wife. In the next chapter we'll see more about how this works out to satisfy both of you.

Spiritual Possession and Oppression

Now that we've touched on Satan's part in our battle against impurity, let's focus on whether sexual impurity represents some form of demon possession.

You aren't possessed by the devil when impurity runs rampant in your life, and you don't need an exorcism. Although it sometimes *feels* like an evil gremlin inside you is driving you to sin, these are merely the compulsions of your bad habits and hormones. You're simply out of control and must bring them all back under the control of your regenerated spirit.

While there's no spiritual *possession* involved, there could be an element of spiritual *oppression*.

FROM FRED: A TURNING POINT

In my case, you be the judge:

Near my six-week mark of going cold turkey, I had a very sensual and violent dream. I was tempted sexually in an extremely enticing manner and yet, for the first time in a dream, I actually said, "No, I won't." (You'll know you're nearing victory when, even in the freedom of your dream state, your subconscious mind still chooses purity.) Then came violent, hand-to-hand combat, and I cried out, "In the name of Jesus, I will defeat you!"

As I said the words "In the name of Jesus," the battle turned in my favor. But when I said the words "I will defeat you," the battle turned violently against me, since I had no power of my own. In desperation, I cried out every name of Jesus I could think of.

Suddenly I awoke, praising God out loud. It was Sunday morning.

Several hours later in church, I worshiped freely all service long for the first time. Praises continued to bubble up out of my heart the rest of the day, that night, and into the next day. For someone who had felt such distance from God for so long, the feeling was glorious.

The explanation? I'm convinced a spiritual oppression in my life was crushed that night, though I can't be dogmatic. I've never been one to look for Satan behind every rock. All I know is that before that night I'd never been able to worship freely. After that night, it flowed easily, and it continues to this day.

Purity Always Brings Spiritual Opposition

While there may not be spiritual oppression involved in your battle, there'll always be spiritual *opposition*. The enemy is constantly near your ear. He doesn't want you to win this fight, and he knows the lies that so often break men's confidence and their will to win. Expect to hear lies and plenty of them.

What we've told you is the truth. There *is* peace and tranquillity for you on the other side of this war. There *is* immeasurable spiritual gain. The deceiver will tell you that Steve Arterburn and Fred Stoeker are crazy, and that you'll soon be as crazy as both of them combined if you follow their ideas.

To help you recognize Satan's lies when you hear them, here's a list of some of them. (After each lie, we'll state the actual truth.)

Satan: "You're the only one dealing with this problem. If anyone ever finds out, you'll be the laughingstock of the church!"

The truth: Most men deal with this problem, so no one will laugh.

Satan: "You failed again. You'll never be able to train your eyes. It's impossible."

The truth: It isn't impossible. Job trained his eyes, didn't he? He was a man just like you.

Satan: "You're being so legalistic! The law is dead and only brings death."

The truth: God still has standards of behavior for us, and you're responsible to live purely by His standards.

Satan: "Oh, c'mon! Don't be such a moron. This 'habit-changing' plan will never work."

The truth: The plan *will* work, because for most men the problem of sexual impurity is nothing more than bad choices evolving into bad habits.

Satan: "Why fight this costly battle when the costs of your impurity are so minimal?"

The truth: You can't always see them, but the costs of your sin are greater than you think.

Satan: "Why live in this high state of alert for the rest of your life? Give up now, and I'll leave you alone."

The truth: Satan just might keep his word and leave you alone, but even if he did, the laws of reaping and sowing would still exact their payment from you. You cannot avoid the costs of sexual impurity. You might as well fight.

Satan: "You'll be awkward in business situations now, especially with women. You won't fit in, and you'll lose business."

The truth: No, you won't be awkward in business situations. You'll be more at ease than ever.

MASTURBATION: A SYMPTOM, NOT THE ROOT

If your sexual impurity includes masturbation, as it does for many men, then some further deceptive tactics from the enemy that you may encounter would include the argument that masturbation is the root of your problem or that it's caused by some psychological pain from your past. Let's tackle these issues head-on.

Let us say it clearly: Masturbation is a symptom of uncontrolled eyes and free-racing thoughts. When you create the new habits of bouncing your eyes and taking thoughts captive, masturbation will cease. Until then, it won't. There's no sense in targeting masturbation itself, because you won't be attacking the real source of the problem. Target the eyes and mind instead.

Listen to Ed Cole, a pastor with a national speaking platform:

> Not only does pornography encourage its readers to create
> an image in their mind, but it also entices them to fantasize
> about it. Usually these fantasies involve an erotic act that

only can be satisfied with someone else or by masturbation. Once an image is created in the mind, that picture actually becomes an idol. The habit of masturbation becomes an act of worshiping that idol. Eventually, it creates a stronghold in the mind and becomes a trap.

Some people think I'm old-fashioned for preaching this, but I continually encounter men who have lost all sense of balance because of habitual masturbation. One man asked, "How many times a day would you consider habitual?" That's reason enough to teach it!

Scripture is silent on the topic of masturbation. Some might even make a case that isolated instances of masturbation to relieve sexual tension are okay, if you're focusing on your wife, not some supermodel, during periods of separation or illness. Wanton masturbation, tied to pornography or whatever gets your motor running, is *always* sin, putting distance between you and God. If you desire holiness, you must stop masturbating. Becoming sexually charged from images other than your wife isn't right.

If you want freedom from masturbation, you must put the ax to the roots. What are the roots? That *you're* stopping short of God's standard, accepting (through your eyes and your mind) more than a hint of immorality in your life.

MASTURBATION AND PSYCHOLOGICAL PAIN

Masturbation is not caused by psychological pain. Some men will argue this point, claiming their masturbation habit isn't rooted in lust but in something entirely less crass. Often that "something" is a constellation of hurt, rejection, and loss of love in their lives caused by a childhood trauma or inept parenting from years past. Do these hurts *cause* masturbation?

Let's take a little true-false test. Which of the following statements are true?

1. Men must *first* deal with the hurt before they can be free from masturbation.

2. Since rejection causes masturbation, rejection and masturbation *must always* coexist together.

3. Masturbation can exist in a man even though he has no impurity of the eyes and mind.

None of these three statements is true. Here's the reality of the situation:

1. It isn't true that you must deal with the hurt first. You can be free from masturbation without ever dealing with the hurt.

2. Rejection and masturbation can each exist in a person's life without the other.

3. Masturbation needs the foreplay of the impure eyes and mind to exist.

"But," you ask, "why do masturbation and psychological pain exist together so often?"

Because of rejection and lost love, men begin to seek for this lost love in all the wrong places. In their search, where's the path of least resistance? A pretend lover, a pornographic lover with a permanent smile. A lover who never says no, one who never rejects. One who never abandons and is always discreet. One who supports the man's ego in the midst of his self-doubt. One who forever says, "Everything will be okay," no matter how high the pressure goes. This path is a chosen path, a path made available by the impure eyes stoking the sexual fever, providing an unending pool of lovers from which to draw.

The reason rejection and masturbation coexist so often is because of our "maleness" and our easy ability to draw true sexual gratification through our eyes. The male eyes give us the *means* to sin broadly and at will. Then, because men get their intimacy from the acts just prior to and during intercourse, masturbation brings a real sense of intimacy and acceptance. This intimacy salves the hurt and rejection. This intimacy is attained easily and without risk, far more easily than at some bar or whorehouse. In fact, it's attained more easily than with a wife, who might say no when you need intimacy most. That's why men choose to masturbate so often.

What if the means to sin are taken away by training the eyes? Masturbation is no longer the path of least resistance. He'll look elsewhere for love. Hopefully, he'll finally deal with the rejection itself. But the masturbation? It goes away. And the hurt manifests itself in some other way. Men aren't victims of masturbation simply because they were victims of emotional trauma. They've chosen it.

Don't be deceived. You can be free from masturbation regardless of past pain.

ACCOUNTABILITY AND YOUR WIFE

As we end this chapter and prepare to focus in part 4 on the first of our three defense perimeters, let's look at a couple of special issues.

The first issue is accountability. For many men who are willing to fight for sexual purity, an important step is finding accountability support in a men's Bible study group, in a smaller group of one or two other men serving as accountability partners, or by going into counseling.

For an accountability partner, enlist a male friend, perhaps someone older and well respected in the church, to encourage you in the heat of battle. The men's ministry at your church can also help you find someone who can pray for you and ask you the tough questions.

Here's how it might go: Let's say Nathan asks for an accountability partner. Ron, a long-time Christian with experience in this area, is asked to help out Nathan. Ron calls Nathan up to chat.

Ron asks, "How's it going, Nathan?" (Both of them know that this refers to masturbation.)

Nathan answers, "I plead the fifth."

"Uh-oh. Talk to me."

"It's been happening every other day for the past two weeks."

"Are you reading the Bible?" Ron asks.

"Yes."

"Are you praying?"

"Yes."

"What's the problem then?"

"Too much TV," Nathan answers. "HBO and *Baywatch* reruns."

Following this conversation, Ron begins contacting Nathan every day because the problem has accelerated and requires more contact. Sometimes Nathan needs to be encouraged. Sometimes he needs to be challenged to do what's right. In the end, though, it comes down to whether Nathan has made a decision to win, a decision for purity. Accountability works only when coupled with a firm commitment to win.

Let us caution you, however, from enlisting your wife as your accountability partner. There's no way most guys will get real with their spouses in something as starkly personal as one's thought life and masturbation habits.

FROM FRED: TELLING YOUR WIFE

That brings up the issue of how much your wife should know about your battle. As your understanding of sexual purity grows, victory will seem possible. With hope rising, perhaps you'll want to tell your wife about your struggle with impurity so that she, your dear, gracious wife, may help you win. But don't be in a big hurry. Remember, our habits are rooted in our maleness. *We* understand them. Women don't. Almost without fail, women who hear about your sexual impurity will think of you as a pervert.

Brenda and I were once discussing the fall of a prominent TV preacher to adultery. "If he were my husband," she stated, "I could not stand to even be around him. He would make me sick!"

Whoa. Brenda doesn't mince words, does she? But the plot quickly turned the next day when she broached the topic again. She told me she was feeling sorry for the disgraced preacher because he'd been desperately struggling alone against a secret sin. Brenda felt that if only his wife had known, she could have helped him through prayer.

"Fred," she said, "if you had such a problem, wouldn't you come to me and tell me? I would want to be praying for you and helping you!"

I burst out laughing. "I couldn't tell you anything like that," I said. "Just yesterday you said you were totally repulsed by it. I'd feel like you wanted me to be cast into a leper colony if you ever knew about such a thing!"

I know some men will disagree with me on this point, and that's fine, because you know your own wife better than I do. But most wives react with shock and revulsion rather than with mercy and prayer.

Besides, how would she respond to you if she knew you had quit the battle, as you'll be tempted to do, especially in the first weeks? Before telling her, you had better check your will to win during the heat of battle. If it will take awhile before you really, really want to win, you'd be better off waiting to tell her, because she'll be watching.

Brenda recently told me that even now, all these years later, she occasionally watches my eyes when we go past billboards, just to check on me. With the good habits in place, I haven't failed her, but who needs that pressure if you aren't ready for it?

Once *you're* absolutely sure that you hate your sin and are ready to change, tell your wife. By this time, she'll suspect something anyway, since your entire sex drive will now be leveled at her.

Having gone through this battle, I know that there are some practical ways a wife can help. First, your wife can be a methadone-like fix when your temperature is rising. Second, when searching for a new sexual equilibrium with her, it obviously helps if she knows what's going on. Third, once your wife understands your eyes, she won't ask you to watch a women's beach volleyball game with her while you're going cold turkey.

RELEASE FOR SINGLES

As a final point, let's explore how the battle plan works in particular for singles. One reason singles can get tripped up in their quest for purity is that they feel overmatched. That's why they're quick to say, "It's easy for you to talk about sexual purity—you're married!" Earlier we dismissed marriage as an adequate answer to purity problems, but the question for singles remains: What are you going to do with the sexual pressure you sometimes feel?

First of all, you have to take by faith that once you get your eyes and mind under control, the sexual pressure will drop off dramatically. You bring most of the sexual pressure onto yourself through visual sensual stimulation and mental fantasy.

Even so, there remains the male seventy-two-hour cycle of sperm production. Without the impurity of the eyes, the pressure generated by lust is gone, but there's still a natural physical pressure for release, though much weaker. "What am I going to do about that?" you might ask. "How will I get release?"

God has supplied the way of release, something with which you're familiar. Clinically it's called "nocturnal emissions." But somewhere in a dank, smelly football locker room, some kid decided to call it a "wet dream," and that name stuck. The good news for singles is that nocturnal emissions can work *for* you in your quest for purity. (They also can work for married guys who aren't as sexually active as they would like to be.)

You may wonder how such dreams will work toward purity. After all, some of these dreams are pretty hot and heavy! But those hot and heavy aspects arise from what *you're* putting into your mind each day. The same pure eyes and mind that keep you from *actively* seeking release during the day will limit the impurity that your mind can use in dreams at night. Even these dreams will be dramatically purer in scope and content.

YOUR GOAL FROM HERE

Now that you've made your decision for sexual purity, you can see more than ever why failing to eliminate every hint of sexual immorality from your life is dangerous. The visual sensuality of immodest dress, movies, commercials, and all the rest will feed your eyes and ignite you sexually. The addictive nature of the chemical responses in your brain's pleasure centers spin tight cords of bondage.

To break those cords, you must cut off the sensual images through your eyes and mind. That's your goal, and the rest of the book is dedicated to showing you how to do it.

Level your sights on the enemy, brother. It's time.

The Heart of a Woman

Once your husband engages in the battle for sexual integrity, here are some things you can pray for him:

1. *Pray that God would keep him from wavering and stumbling.* Ask God to put more light on his path and more courage in his step.
2. *Pray against spiritual opposition in the form of lies.* As you know, Satan will lie to him to weaken his will to win. Pray that Satan's efforts to confuse him will be ineffective.

3. *Pray against possible spiritual oppression.* Ask God to release power to break any spiritual oppression over your lives and your home that has resulted from his sexual sin.

Along with prayer, there are other ways you can help him win this battle. Once he tells you he's going cold turkey, be like a merciful vial of methadone for him. Increase your availability to him sexually, though this may be difficult for you since your husband might have told you some things that repulse you. Since your sex drive, as a woman, is tied to relationship, you may feel betrayed, just as if your husband had an actual affair.

It may help you to view this from a male's perspective, where "relationship" and "sex" do not have such a tight bond. Please don't misunderstand us. His lusting was definitely a moral betrayal, but it wasn't necessarily a betrayal of the heart. You may still be his one and only true love, the one he could never, ever leave. He has a fractional addiction to the chemical high, but don't assume his heart for you is untrue. Mercy is probably your best tack—with accountability, of course.

On another issue: Do you believe that God has given you, as a wife, a responsibility to be a role model of godliness and holiness to your husband? We received some interesting comments to this question.

Some women don't feel modeling godliness for their husbands is their role at all. Cathy said, "My responsibility is to love him, and that will manifest itself in godliness. But I feel the role model responsibility is primarily his, since he's the leader of our home."

We don't disagree with Cathy's last statement, but we want to point out that since you're one flesh with your husband, you have a right, even a duty, to play such a role as well.

If a wife acts as a role model, how should it look in everyday life?

Heather said, "My first responsibility as a role model is to be pure and true sexually to my husband, as I expect him to be."

Wendy said, "I don't try to get Mark to do things that we both know are wrong, like watching sensual movies," she said. "I don't do things that would be a stumbling block to him, like leaving Victoria's Secret catalogs lying around open."

Many women feel that they care more about godliness than their husbands do. (As men, this is to our shame.) Andrea said, "Lately, through the preaching of several men and a worship conference a year ago, I met God in a new way and have changed more in the past year than ever before. God has given me a deep desire to purify my life and my home. It's been frustrating at times, though, because there have been many things I've wanted to change, but I've met resistance from my husband. He's a wonderful Christian, but in talking with my sister recently, we've concluded there's a tendency among men to brush off women's attempts to purify our homes. For example, I'm no longer comfortable with certain movies. I don't like to watch them, nor do I like my children to watch them. But rather than come across as a holier-than-thou person, God has helped me to keep my mouth shut after voicing my concerns and instead pray about the situation and to pray for my husband."

Cathy added, "I've never felt I *cared* more about holiness than my husband, but I think I put more *energy* into it. Maybe it comes more easily to a woman; I don't know. If he seems to be struggling in a certain area, if I confront him or try to be a leader, it has much less effect than when I pray and fast for him."

PART IV

victory with
your eyes

bouncing the eyes

To set up your first defense perimeter with your eyes, you want to employ the strategies of *bouncing* your eyes and *starving* your eyes as well as the tactic of taking up a "sword" and a "shield."

Let's first consider bouncing. You can win this battle by training your eyes to "bounce" away from sights of pretty women and sensual images. If you "bounce your eyes" for six weeks, you can win this war.

The problem is that your eyes have always bounced toward the sexual, and you've made no attempt to end this habit. To combat it, you need to build a reflex action by training your eyes to immediately bounce away from the sexual, like the jerk of your hand away from a hot stove.

Let's repeat that, for emphasis: When your eyes bounce toward a woman, they must bounce away *immediately.*

But why must the bounce be immediate? After all, you might argue, a glance isn't the same as lusting.

If we define "lusting" as staring open-mouthed until drool pools at your feet, then a glance isn't the same as lusting. But if we define lusting as any look that creates that little chemical high, that little pop, then we have something a bit more difficult to measure. This chemical high happens more quickly than you realize.

In our experience, drawing the line at "immediate" is clean and easy for the mind and eyes to understand. This "line in the sand" seems to work effectively.

So how do we train this new bouncing reflex?

For openers, the habit of what your eyes look at is no different from any other habit. Since experts say that anything done consistently for twenty-one days becomes a new habit, you must find some way to *consistently* bounce your eyes over time.

YOUR TACTICS

When you start bouncing your eyes, your body will fight against you in peculiar, unexpected ways. Sexual sin has an addictive nature, and your body will not want to give up on its pleasures. You'll have to creatively respond in your quest for purity, and you do that through these two logical steps:

1. Study yourself. How and where are you attacked most?
2. Define your defense for each of the greatest enemies you've identified.

Your first step is listing your own "greatest enemies." What are the most obvious and prolific sources of sensual images apart from your wife? Where do you look most often? Where are you weakest?

FROM FRED: MY GREATEST ENEMIES

I had no problem coming up with a list of my six biggest areas of weakness.

1. lingerie advertisements
2. female joggers in tight nylon shorts
3. billboards showing scantily clad women
4. beer-and-bikini commercials
5. movies rated PG-13 or higher
6. receptionists with low-cut or tight blouses

What are your main areas of weakness? In choosing them, remember that they must be areas from which you *visually* draw sexual satisfaction.

Some make the mistake of choosing nonvisual weaknesses for this list. For instance, Justin initially included the following three on his list:

1. Showers.
2. Being home alone.
3. Working late.

We can all understand why these are troublesome. In the shower, you're nude with warm water cascading down your body. When you're home alone, no one is around to discover you. When working late, you feel sorry for yourself and need "comfort."

But such weak spots needn't be targeted if you train your eyes to bounce and eliminate the visual stimuli. With no food for the mental fancies, the sexual fever that draws your mind to sin in these situations will be broken. These situations will lose their power naturally.

DEFINING YOUR DEFENSES

I can't define the best defense for your weaknesses, but let me share mine so you'll get a feel for the process.

Lingerie Ads

Lingerie advertisements were my worst enemy and remained difficult to control for quite some time. I was successfully bouncing my eyes in every other area long before I had total victory here. Why? Those ad inserts were the most sexually satisfying images of them all, and from time to time, I hit the mother lode: a swimsuit feature or an exercise feature illustrated with bun-fitting spandex all around.

Not only did I train my eyes to bounce away from such print ads, I also trained myself not to pick them up in the first place. My defense was to establish a number of rules to keep these images out of my hands before my eyes had a chance to see them.

Rule 1: When my hand reached for a magazine or insert, if I sensed in even the slightest way that my underlying motive was to see something sensual, I forfeited my right to pick up that magazine or insert. Forever.

To be honest, this didn't work well at first. Even though sensing my motive was easy, forfeiting my right to pick it up was not. My flesh simply ignored my spirit, shouting, "Shut up! I want this, and I'll have it!" My flesh won time after time, but as I began to succeed in the other five areas, my hatred for the sin grew, and as it grew, my will and discipline grew stronger. I never gave up, and the lingerie ads finally failed to ensnare me.

Rule 2: If a magazine had an overtly sensual female on the cover, I tore off the cover and threw it away.

Mail-order clothing catalogs or swimsuit magazines with sensual cover pictures can sit on your coffee table, drawing your eyes all month long. Now, I ask you this: What if a full-breasted woman in a teensy-weensy teensy bikini came to your home and sat down on your coffee table and said, "I'll just sit here awhile, but I promise to leave by the end of the month"? Would you let her stay to catch your eye every time you walked in the room? I don't think so. So why do you leave her there in picture form?

Once I remember Brenda asking, "What's been happening to all our magazine covers?" But that's how I handled the problem, and today she happily grants me full censorship rights!

Rule 3: If I was genuinely looking for sale prices on camping equipment or tools in department store inserts, I would allow myself to pick up the insert but I forced myself to start looking from the back.

Don't ask me how I know, but the lingerie ads are usually found on pages two and three. The camping, automotive, and tool ads are on the last pages. By opening the insert from the rear, I avoided seeing the young models entirely. When a sensual image snuck up on me even though my motives for leafing through a magazine were proper, I kept the normal covenant to bounce my eyes *immediately.*

Female Joggers

Whenever I approached a roadside jogger while driving my car, my eyes fixed on her, appreciating her beauty, just as Steve did with the Malibu jogger in the first chapter. But trying to look away from a jogger creates a problem: I'd have to look completely away from the road not to see her. That's driving dangerously, even in Iowa! After all, I didn't want to run anyone over.

Studying the situation, I found a solution. Rather than look completely away, I could look to the opposite side of the road. I discovered that it was impossible to lust with only my peripheral vision, so I used this to my advantage.

My body began to fight back in some interesting ways. First, my brain argued fiercely with me: *If you keep this up, you'll cause a wreck.* I considered his argument, then answered, *You know and I know that's highly unlikely.*

My body's second attempt to stop me was very peculiar. Whenever I saw a jogger and reflexively looked away, my mind would trick me into believing I recognized the individual, prompting a second look. My mind was so good at this that nearly every female jogger I saw reminded me of someone I knew. You talk about irritating! It took awhile for me to stop falling for that deception.

My brain tried another trick. As I passed the jogger without a direct look, I would momentarily relax. In the same moment, my brain took advantage of my lowered guard by ordering my eyes to glance into the rearview mirror for a more direct look. That really burned me up! I had to learn not to drop my guard after passing, and in time that trick faded away as well.

Whenever I was taken in by one of these tricks, I'd bark to myself in sharp rebuke, "You've made a covenant with your eyes! You can't do that anymore." In the first two weeks, I must have said it a million times, but the repeated confession of truth eventually worked a transformation in me.

Billboards

Billboards are notorious for featuring some long, tall, slinky, sexy woman who seems to whisper, "C'mon, big boy, buy this stuff and you'll get me, too!" I know of one giant billboard for a rock radio station that showed a closeup of bikini-clad breasts with this tag line: "What a pair!"

My defense mechanism, of course, was to bounce my eyes, but I took it a step further by remembering where the sensual billboards were placed along my commute. That way I ensured myself that I wouldn't drive up to them each day without thinking and get tomahawked.

When designing my defense against billboards, I thought of my experience in high school driving a hotel van. We had a contract with the airlines to drive pilots and flight attendants from the airport to the hotel. The contract required that we complete the trip within ten minutes. Only one route from the airport was short enough to make the time limit—an unpaved road with a billion potholes. I painfully learned of the direct correlation between the number of potholes I hit and the size of my tip. So I methodically memorized every pothole on that road and the driving angles necessary to miss most of them. Eventually, I could practically drive that road blindfolded and hit very few potholes.

With the billboards, it's always easier for me to memorize their locations and to avoid visual contact entirely rather than looking and then bouncing my eyes.

Beer-and-Bikini Commercials

A red-blooded American male can't watch a major sporting event without being assaulted by commercials showing a bunch of half-naked women cavorting on some beach with some beer-soaked yahoos. What's a man to do?

The answer is to maintain control of the remote and zap those commercials! The defense is simple: All sexy women get zapped by the clicker.

Phasers set to kill, Spock. This is the best way. You can hit another station and come back in sixty seconds. (This approach gives you another reason to keep the clicker away from the wife and kids.)

As your children watch you click away, you serve as a living example of godliness in your home, and that will speak volumes to them.

Movies

We have a very good rule at home. Any video unsuitable for the kids is probably unsuitable for adults. With this rule in place, sensual movies have never been a problem in our home.

Not watching randy movies is more difficult when you're on the road and in a hotel room all by yourself. Still, a Christian lives like a Christian when no one else is around, including when you're in a hotel room on a business trip.

Do you remember the transport device in *Star Trek* that made the phrase "Beam me up, Scotty!" part of the cultural lexicon? You want to say honestly that while you're on any business trip, your wife could "beam into" your hotel room at any moment and never find you watching something improper.

With that standard, I would have been busted repeatedly earlier in my life. Once five o'clock came and the business day was over, I had hours with nothing to do. This left me very vulnerable to watching cable movies, and I fell for them again and again.

In defense, I set some rules. I tried a variation of my "motive rule" with magazines. When I reached for the clicker to turn it on, I would check my motives. If they were clean, I would allow myself to turn on the TV, usually sticking with the news or ESPN. Trouble was, I would get bored and, without thinking, start channel surfing.

The "motive rule" worked better with magazines, because once I forfeited the right to look at them, I could get up and go elsewhere and forget about them. Not so with the hotel room TV; I still had hours alone in the room with the blank screen staring back at me, tempting me.

So I grounded myself from hotel TV. I decided that I'd lost my privileges and wasn't allowed to turn it on for a while. Sound drastic? I've had some men tell me that they put blankets over their TVs to keep them out of sight. Others call the front desk and ask them to "block" the pay-per-view soft-core movies. Whatever you have to do, do it.

Receptionists

Sometimes when I enter office buildings, the receptionist might be standing upon my arrival. Telling her my name, she would then bend over to the phone to announce my arrival. Often her loose-fitting, silky blouse fell open to reveal everything. It had never occurred to me to turn away; I simply figured it was my lucky day.

When I began my search for purity, this had to stop. The defense was simple. Before, when I came in and saw the receptionist standing, I knew what might happen and looked for it. Now I use this same knowledge to my advantage. When I see her standing, I avert my eyes even before she bends over. Or if I see her walking toward a file cabinet, I avert my eyes before she bends over for that file, leaving me that nice view of her rear end. Of all the weaknesses, this one was addressed most easily. I now naturally turn away.

A Word on Technological Temptations

I want to touch on three stories that I've run across since *Every Man's Battle* first released in 2000.

First, consider Brady, who'd been dealing with lust and pornography for some time until he read our book. He'd learned to begin treating women respectfully with his eyes and mind and to see them as people instead of as hot collections of interesting body parts. "I was doing great, and I wasn't even thinking about girls in that way, at least until the day I was in a chat room online and the chat turned sexy. Then I noticed the Web cam that my dad had purchased. The next thing I knew, I was broadcasting myself to five girls while masturbating. When I was done, I felt so bad that I cried my eyes out, but the next day, I did the very same thing. By now it's like I'm addicted to doing that stuff. I hate what I do, but somehow I can't seem to stop."

Next, there's Craig, who met nineteen-year-old Clara over the Internet. Because Craig was a twenty-seven-year-old single missionary, Clara immediately put 100 percent stock in his character. Their cell-phone conversations lingered until the early hours of the morning. For many weeks their talks centered on spiritual matters such as, "When is Jesus returning?" and, "What will heaven be like?" But after those conversations grew stale, the topics turned more personal: "What would we do if we were alone together right now?" or, "What turns you on most?"

One night Craig, feeling relatively sure that Clara wouldn't deny his request, asked her to use her cell phone to make a video clip of herself masturbating. Clara thought it was the least she could do to satisfy them both what with all the miles separating them. But after that deed was done, they were eaten up by guilty consciences. They vowed not to do it again—a promise that lasted all of two weeks. Even as "technical virgins," they were both hooked on phone sex...until Clara's mom found her phone and the most recent videos sent. But those consequences were minimal compared to what happened to Jennifer.

Jennifer was excited to land a new job as a youth pastor at her church. But before starting the position, she went on a Caribbean cruise with a friend. That's where Jennifer met Jack, a guy who thought she was the most stunning woman aboard. The only catch was that Jack was married, and so was Jennifer. Even so, they exchanged cell phone numbers. Within weeks an occasional chat became frequent calls, and they exchanged text messages with language so steamy you could fry an egg on Jennifer's cell phone. When she mentioned wearing Victoria's Secret underwear, Jack pestered her to send intimate photos. She figured that as long as the two of them never did anything physical, then they weren't *really* being unfaithful to their spouses.

Obviously, Jack's wife didn't agree. Imagine Jennifer's horror when her pastor (and boss) called her into his office, then showed her an e-mail Jack's wife had sent detailing many of these text messages with the sexy photos attached. The first paragraph of the e-mail explained, "I've had a private investigator following my husband around for months, and I think you deserve to know what your youth pastor has been up to."

The scorned wife also copied every staff member in the online church directory. Jennifer lost her job, not to mention her husband's trust, and she is going through counseling to try and put the pieces of her life back together.

I share these stories with you because there's a common thread: these people all compromised their sexual integrity, and as a result they were publicly humiliated. But it's not the Web cams or cell phones or broadband technology that are at fault; it's how these people were behaving in the first place that got them into trouble. To avoid similar problems, consider these six guidelines:

1. Hot conversation, whether by phone or by text or by computer, gets your mind racing and puts your body in the lead. Since this talk takes you from one level of arousal to the next, it's not "sophisticated" or just "harmless fun." It's foreplay, and it works on the pleasure centers of the brain exactly like porn. Why else would 1-900 numbers be so profitable?

2. When the next new technology comes along and you wonder if what you're doing is right, ask these questions: *Does it drive me from one level of arousal to the next? Am I driven to do it again and again?* If so, call it what it is—sex outside of marriage. Remember, you don't have to be with someone to have sex. We call it phone sex because we get the same kick and the same high as other forms of sex, whether we're in her presence or not.

3. It's none of your business what turns her on unless you've entered into a covenant relationship with her in marriage. Ever.

4. When it comes to any form of text messages (cell phones, e-mails, Facebook, and so on), don't type anything that you wouldn't want someone—like your wife or your pastor—to read or hear you say in person.

5. The fastest way to put a stop to text messages with inappropriate language or innuendos is to simply not respond. Let the other person eat static. If she follows up with a "why aren't you responding?" message, then you can reply with something like, "I don't play that game."

6. If you're married, you have no business texting her, e-mailing her, or calling her at all. If you must contact a married woman, communicate through her husband.

When you consider how you'll use any communication technology, remember these three stories. Think about such a possible disaster like you think of an STD: something that can only happen when you mix sex with irresponsibility. Remember, too, that a picture is worth a thousand words. Never, ever create sexual photos, videos, e-mails, text messages, or anything else that someone could keep and share in the future.

starving the eyes

As you set up your defense perimeter with your eyes, a further strategic approach is to think of *starving* the eyes.

Remember again our definition for sexual purity: *You are sexually pure when no sexual gratification comes from anyone or anything but your wife.* Our battle centers on our sexual gratification.

Let's picture that gratification in another way. As a man, you need a certain amount of food and water to live. The amounts differ for each of us, based upon genetics, metabolism, and activity. It's even possible to suspend these needs for a while, as when fasting or limiting your food intake to lose weight.

Similarly, you require a certain amount of sexual gratification. Your sex drive may be suspended by God with a gift of abstinence. And you can adjust the required volume of sexual gratification to some extent. By controlling the sexual images entering your eyes and mind, your system may become used to living on less, but in the end, you still have a certain volume of sexual gratification you need to fill.

BOWLS OF GRATIFICATION

Unfortunately, there's no unit of measure for sexual gratification, like liters or inches. But we're going to make one up, and we'll call them "bowls." Imagine that your current level of sexual hunger requires ten bowls of sexual gratification per week. These bowls of gratification *should* be filled from your single legitimate vessel, the wife whom God provided for you. But because males soak up sexual gratification through the eyes, we can effortlessly fill our bowls from other sources.

Our sensualized culture pours sexual imagery freely with the potential to fill our bowls continually and forever. Our eyes can feast away! If your sexual need is ten bowls a week, you can easily draw five bowls from the culture, while drawing only five from your wife. (That's not the same as having intercourse five times a week, because we can draw sexual gratification from our wives in many ways.)

While this "bowls" imagery oversimplifies the details, it clarifies the process involved in our sexual gratification.

STARVING THE EYES

To attain sexual purity as we defined it, we must starve our eyes of the bowls of sexual gratification that come from outside our marriage. When you starve your eyes and eliminate "junk sex" from your life, you'll deeply crave "real food"—your wife. And no wonder. She's the only thing in the cupboard, and you're hungry!

This newfound hunger will shock her. She has been accustomed to providing you five bowls a week, primarily through physical foreplay and sexual intercourse. Things were at equilibrium. Suddenly you need an extra five bowls from her. For no apparent reason, you come calling for intercourse twice as often.

If this were all there was to it, it wouldn't seem so mysterious. To women, men *always* want more sex than they're getting! But there's more to it. Since your visual gratification now pours only from her, she's looking *very* good to you. Perhaps you haven't looked at her quite like this since you were newlyweds. While this sensation is vaguely pleasant to her, it can also be a tad jarring. *Has he been taking aphrodisiacs?* she wonders. She doesn't quite know what to do, except to send you outside to play with the kids while she undresses in the master bathroom.

And it's not just the *looking.* Once you're winning the battle, you'll be saying things you haven't uttered for years like, "I can't wait for tonight, baby." All your imaginative creativity now blossoms upon your marriage bed, not in some fantasy world. You'll be fully enamored with her!

Again, this is vaguely pleasant to her, but she's also troubled. *Where are these new ideas coming from?* she may wonder. *Has he been having an affair? What's going on?*

She'll probably ask you what's going on, and once she learns what's cooking, you'll both need to find a new sexual equilibrium. The extra five bowls from outside the marriage must now be provided from inside the marriage.

FROM FRED: PUTTING UP WITH ME

After I'd gone cold turkey on sexual images for about three weeks, I remember vividly how Brenda noticed the geometric rise in my desire for her. Constantly telling her how beautiful she looked, I was all over her, patting her, hugging her, touching her. I also was desiring intercourse far more often, and as the new higher pace continued, it dawned upon Brenda that this might not be just some simple jag or a phase.

She panicked, blurting out, "What am I doing to make myself so attractive? I have to stop it!"

That moment was hilarious. I told her what was going on and that I couldn't really help my heightened desire for her. "All my desires are coming straight at you, and I don't quite know what to do about it yet. I promise I'll work hard to get back to an equilibrium that we both can live with." Brenda didn't know whether to be relieved or shocked, but she expressed a willingness to allow me time to find that equilibrium—and to put up with me until then.

Those days revealed to me just how much I'd been stealing from Brenda by watching sensuous R-rated movies and inspecting the lingerie catalogs. Those things provide far more sexual gratification than we might expect, although Satan would have you think otherwise.

When a fellow named Tom heard me speak about removing every hint of sexual sin from our lives, he said, "I think you're defining sexual sin much too broadly when you include movies, ad inserts, joggers, and the rest. These are nothing!"

I disagreed. I was evidently drawing so much sexual gratification from these "innocuous" sources that, once they were removed and the whole sexual burden was placed upon Brenda, she felt it. Eventually, my sex drive was retooled to live within God's boundaries, but it didn't happen until I went cold turkey on depriving myself of impure sexual images.

ADJUSTING TO PURITY

After going cold turkey, I found that my required bowls of gratification didn't come entirely from increased frequency of sexual intercourse. Some bowls came visually, but only through Brenda. The balance came from a natural downward adjustment of my sexual hunger, maybe dropping from ten bowls to eight bowls a week as I adjusted to my new sexual purity.

"Wait a minute, Fred," you say. "Cutting down from ten bowls to eight bowls seems unfair. I'm being cheated, all because I'm obeying God!"

I guarantee you won't feel cheated. With your whole sexual being now focused upon your wife, sex with her will be so transformed that your satisfaction will explode off any known scale. Yes, even while consuming fewer bowls. It's a personal guarantee, backed by the full faith, credit, and authority of the Word of God.

STILL BEAUTIFUL

We think Randy's story can help deepen your understanding of this paradox. Speaking of his wife, Regina, he told us, "Things got to the point that she just didn't excite me anymore. What with the chaos of parenting and year after year of being responsible for the kids, Regina had become just a good, trusted friend. She always came through in the clutch, but like any good friend, I didn't particularly find her sexy.

"Then one day I was making a delivery in a building downtown and, rounding a corner, I came face to face with a goddess. Young with long, rich black hair. Long legs in heels, and full breasts crowning a silky-thin, miniskirt sundress. I actually gasped out loud. It was totally embarrassing. My chest heaved, and my mouth instantly went bone dry. I may or may not have staggered; I don't know. But I felt as if I'd been knocked cold.

"From time to time over the next few days, I got to thinking about Regina as I drove around at work. My wife had never been jaw-dropping beautiful, even when younger. I remembered, though, that when I first laid eyes on her, she was *very* striking to me and blew all my whistles! I wondered, *Was she still beautiful to me?*

"One night, as I watched her prepare dinner for us, I noticed that she was still quite pretty. She was a bit heavier, and her rear end hung a little, as did the skin around her eyes and neck. But she *was* pretty to me. Why didn't I appreciate her beauty anymore?

"Shortly after that, I heard Fred speak about starving the eyes. I'd never been in gross sexual sin, but I'd never really guarded my eyes either. I watched any movies I wanted, and I often looked a little too long at the younger girls at work, but I really didn't think these things affected my life. But after Fred's talk, I began to wonder. I paid more attention to my eyes, and I found that they were collecting a lot more sexual gratification than I'd thought.

"Thinking maybe that was why I'd lost my appetite for Regina, I began starving my eyes. I couldn't believe what happened! Regina is no longer just a friend. She's become a goddess, at least to me. And it's funny—the more I draw only from her, the more my tastes change. Those little rolls of fat on her back and sides used to bother me. Now, as I run my finger over them, they actually turn me on. Isn't that crazy? And that little bit of rear end that hangs below her underwear? Before, it only emphasized to me how much weight she'd gained. Now, that little piece just explodes my desire for her. Regina may not be a supermodel, but I'm no day at the beach either. Yet to me, she's like Miss America now."

THE SEXUAL PAYOFF

The magazines at the supermarket checkout might say, "Fantasize to a Better Sex Life." The talk shows may say, "Let variety improve your sex life—adultery can be good!" But in God's kingdom, obedience always ends in joy, peace, and in this case, thrills.

You can count on a sexual payoff from obedience. Whether your wife is wide or narrow or lumpy or smooth, when you focus your full attention on "your fountain," she'll become ever more beautiful to you. Her weak points will become sexy because they're yours and yours alone. They're all you have, and you can cherish them and let them fulfill you.

Maybe this shouldn't surprise us so much. After all, standards of beauty are not fixed. In centuries past, the great master painters depicted heavy, rounded women as the ultimate beauty. In the 1920s, thin, flat-chested women reigned. In the 1960s, the full-breasted, voluptuous girls were queen. In the 1980s and 1990s, muscled, glistening athletic women ignited us. Men adapt to each time period, their tastes formed by what they view, and the same will happen in this new millennium.

If you limit your eyes to your wife only, your own tastes will adapt to what you're viewing. Your wife's strengths *and* weaknesses will become your tastes. Eventually, she'll be beyond comparison in your eyes.

your sword and shield

These strategies for bouncing and starving the eyes may sound rather simple. Maybe even easy to do. But they aren't. Satan fights you with lies, while your body fights you with the desires and strength of deeply entrenched bad habits. To win, you need a sword and a shield. Of all the parts of your battle plan, this is likely the most important.

YOUR SWORD

You'll need a good Bible verse to use as a sword and rallying point.

Just one? It may be useful to memorize several verses of Scripture about purity, as they work to eventually transform and wash the mind. But in the cold-turkey, day-to-day fight against impurity, having several memory verses might be as cumbersome as strapping on a hundred-pound backpack to engage in hand-to-hand combat. You aren't agile enough.

That's why we recommend a single "attack verse," and it better be quick. We suggest the opening line of Job 31:

I have made a covenant with my eyes.

When you fail and look at a jogger, say sharply, "No, I've made a covenant with my eyes. I can't do that!" When you look at a busty billboard, say, "No, I've made a covenant with my eyes. I can't do that!" This action will be a quick dagger to the heart of your enemy.

YOUR SHIELD

Your shield—a protective verse that you can reflect on and draw strength from even when you aren't in the direct heat of battle—may be even more important than your sword, because it places temptation out of earshot.

We suggest selecting this verse as your shield:

> Flee from sexual immorality.... You are not your own; you were bought at a price. Therefore honor God with your body. (1 Corinthians 6:18-20)

We've distilled this shield-verse to its core kernel, and repeated it in the face of many tempting situations when facing sensual images or thoughts:

You have no right to look at that or think about it. You haven't the authority.

A shield such as this will help you think rightly about the real issues involved as you face temptation in your fight for purity. Satan's power of temptation lies in your supposed right to make decisions regarding your behavior. If you didn't believe you had that right, no tempting power could touch you.

FROM FRED: LOOKING AT PLAYBOY

Once on an overnight hotel stay, I walked down the hallway to the ice machine. On top of the machine was a *Playboy* magazine. Believing I had a right to choose my behavior, I asked myself this question: Should I look at this *Playboy* or not?

The moment I asked that question, I opened myself to counsel. I began talking pros and cons to myself. But far worse, I opened myself to Satan's counsel. He wanted to be heard on this issue.

He cajoled and lied, keeping my mind focused on the conversation so I didn't even notice my body slipping down the slope of lust. By the time he finished, the only answer I wanted to hear was "Yes, you should look at it."

Therein lies the power of temptation. You may fear that temptation will be too strong for you in this battle, but temptations honestly have no power at all without our own arrogant questions.

Put yourself in my situation that night. Away from home on a business trip, you're walking to fill your ice bucket and you spy the *Playboy* magazine. But your mind has been thinking on your shield-verse, the words from 1 Corinthians 6.

What's your internal response now?

I have no right to even consider looking at it. I haven't the authority.

That conviction leaves no room for pros and cons to drift deceitfully about your brain. And as for Satan, since you asked no questions, no conversation with him transpires—a conversation in which he could try to get you to change your mind.

FOR THE MIND AS WELL AS THE EYES

Your sword and shield will help strengthen you not only in controlling your eyes, but also as you establish a defense perimeter with your mind (which we'll explore thoroughly in part 5).

Here's an example. You're driving down some freeway on the way to an appointment. You and your wife have had some distance between you for a few weeks. Suddenly an old girlfriend pops into your mind. Note the great difference in perspective between the following two possible responses:

1. Should I daydream about my old girlfriend right now?
2. I don't even have the right to ask such a question, because I don't have the authority to make that decision.

The first response implies that you have the authority and the right to make that decision. The second implies that the question itself is moot.

We call this second response *living within our rights*. If we live within our rights, God's laws of reaping and sowing protect us. Once we step beyond our rights, the sowing and reaping laws work against us. We're in mutiny, having stolen authority from our Captain. And we're back within earshot of Satan.

Ray was confused recently about his rights. "My wife, Jan, and I had a big fight the other day," he said. "I was looking at some pretty women and gave a little whistle. She got angry and said I shouldn't be looking at other women. Well, I think it's okay to look at other women. Just because I can't order doesn't mean I can't look at the menu."

Our response: First of all, we don't think married men have the biblical right to look at other women. But once a wife says she's bothered by it, all rights surely vanish. Ray stepped outside his rights when he thought he could look at other women like an epicure regarding the menu of a fine restaurant. He opened himself up to Satan's confusing counsel. Here's what he may have whispered:

1. "God made them beautiful on purpose. Of course you should look. He intended that for you!"
2. "It won't hurt anything…you're only looking. You aren't really lusting yet."
3. "Life is unbearable to live by such tight standards. God could not possibly have intended that for you. Go ahead and look. He loves you and wants you to live life more abundantly."

4. "I know your wife is bothered when you look at other women, but she's immature. *She* has the problem, not you! She needs to grow in knowledge and freedom. Jealousy is a sin, and she obviously has a sin problem."

Outside his rights and with his shield down, Ray was nodding his head to all four statements.

But it didn't have to happen.

Shield yourself from the power of temptation by submitting to God's definition of your rights.

FROM FRED: WHAT TO EXPECT

Okay, you've made a covenant with your eyes to starve them and to train them to bounce. Maybe you've defined your weak areas, creating a custom defense for each one, and have picked up your sword and shield. What can you expect to happen over the next few weeks, even years?

Here's a bit of the time line that unfolded for me as my perimeters went up.

Short-term results: The first two weeks were largely failure after failure for me. My eyes simply would not fall in line and bounce away from the sexual. My shields from Satan's lies were weak, but I kept plodding ahead in faith, knowing God was with me in this.

During the third and fourth weeks, hope dawned as I began to win about as often as I failed. I can't overemphasize how dramatic and surprising this change was for me. God's blessings and gifts truly go beyond what we can ask or think, for when we sow righteousness, only the mind of God can conceive of the blessings we'll reap. I couldn't believe how much I now lived to please Brenda.

During the fifth and sixth weeks, my eyes found a consistency in bouncing away from the sensual. At the end of the sixth week I had the intense dream I spoke of earlier. The spiritual oppression lifted, and the veil of distance from God vanished. Though I was still not perfect, the rest was downhill.

For you, it needn't take long to raise the defense perimeter of your eyes. If you really want it, it comes quickly. More than once, men have said to me, "Fred, this is amazing, but it happened just like you said! Right about the sixth week, it all came together!" But six weeks is surely no hard-and-fast rule. It may take less time or perhaps more, depending on your strongholds and your commitment to the task at hand.

Long-term results: As you keep living purely, the hedge of protection from temptation grows thicker around you. If you're diligent, it becomes a much longer throw for Satan to lob temptation grenades into your living quarters.

In the long term, do you still have to monitor your eyes? Yes, because the natural bent of your eyes is to sin, and you'll return to bad habits if you're careless. But with only the slightest effort, good habits are permanent.

On a practical note, if you live in a four-season region, late spring and early summer calls for a fresh dose of diligence as warmer temperatures allow women to wear less clothing. Plan to heighten your defenses at those times.

After a year or so—though it may take longer—nearly all major skirmishes will stop. Bouncing your eyes will become deeply entrenched. Your brain, now policing itself tightly, will rarely slip anymore, having given up long ago on its chances to return to the old days of pornographic pleasure highs.

SLIGHTLY CRAZY?

Looking back at the details of our plan, even we will admit that it all sounds slightly crazy. Defenses, brain tricks, bouncing your eyes, forfeiting rights. Man! We wonder if even Job would be a bit startled.

On the other hand, maybe we should expect a sound plan to look this way. Consider all the men who are called to purity, yet so few seem to know how to do it.

What's the bottom line? It took all our resources and creativity to destroy the old habits and every inch of freedom in Christ to walk free from sin. We had been owned by these habits for years, taking whatever women we desired with our eyes.

Freedom from sin is worth dying for, according to Jesus. Take it from us…it's also worth living for!

The Heart of a Woman

As you look to help your husband in his battle for his eyes, don't look through your woman's eyes. Your sexuality is *relational,* so you'll assume you're part of the problem, but he has an eye problem that probably has nothing to do with you.

A story about Terry and Courtney can illustrate this point. Now married, they met while attending Bible school together. Courtney is a very beautiful woman. (The joke on campus was that Courtney averaged one marriage proposal per week.) That means that after Terry married her, his eyes should have never strayed, right?

No, his eyes did stray. Was there something wrong with the relationship? No. Did Courtney lose her beauty? No. What was the problem then? Terry's eyes and mind were untrained. His problem had nothing to do with Courtney.

If a husband has a problem with his eyes, his wife often puts useless pressure on herself to improve her looks or to go out of her way to do nice things for him, thinking it will help stop the problem. "I thought I had to make myself look nice for my husband," Heather said. "I thought I should be giving him backrubs, sitting down and talking to him, and really listening when he came home." Such things won't change her husband's eye problem, however, if he has one.

Men certainly will appreciate your efforts to look your best. Andrea said, "I do my part to make sure he has no reason to have wandering eyes. Even if I'm just home all day with nowhere to go, I still do my hair and makeup and wear nice clothes."

But if a man has eye problems, it *isn't* because his wife needs to look more enticing. "For the most part," Brenda said, "it seems that it's the husband's job to be pure. I don't really see a lot in this chapter that relates to women. We can't control joggers, receptionists, or billboards. This is mostly stuff that men must handle on their own. It's more their battle than ours."

Your husband won't complain if you try to look nice. And as you seek to help, here are some other useful ideas:

1. Watch what he watches. Let's say it's a quiet Saturday night, and you and the kids decide that an evening of watching professional figure skating is the perfect family-night activity. You've settled in with popcorn, and your daughter's eyes are aglow with anticipation.

Your husband may find at this time that viewing female skater after skater in next-to-nothing outfits is too much. If he begs off and wants to putter around in the garage, let him.

2. Help him find the new equilibrium. When he goes cold turkey and his hunger for you escalates, help him without complaint. *Does this mean I have to dance around like some saloon girl?* No. You needn't wear leather and chains, nor take a yogurt bath with him. He just has a heightened hunger for you. Simply meet it with a caring, respectful softness and willingness until an equilibrium is found.

3. Defuse the seventy-two-hour cycle. As we mentioned before, when men aren't getting regular sexual release, their eyes are more difficult to control. Help him out in this battle. Give him release.

Does that mean he should have sex anytime he wants? Of course not. The Bible says you should not withhold sex for long periods of time, but men love to interpret that scripture incorrectly by saying they have a right to intercourse as often as they want. We've heard stories about some husbands who coerced their wives into sexual intercourse one, two, and sometimes three times a day!

Perhaps your husband needs to be reminded that it's a seventy-two-*hour* cycle, not a seventy-two-*minute* cycle! If your husband is demanding sex more than once a day, he likely has a lust problem that needs to be dealt with or he's a borderline sex addict who needs therapy.

4. *Allow him to ogle you a bit.* Let him see you come out of the shower naked. If he can no longer be drawn elsewhere visually, let him draw from you. You may not care much for your own body and you may not want to be ogled, but you'll be looking better and better to him.

5. *Do regular checkups.* As we've said before, you're not to be his account-ability partner, but checking up on him—with humor and grace—helps him while also encouraging you and making you feel more secure. "When we're driving along," Cathy said, "and we come up on some lady jogging in black tights, I probe a little deeper to see what his reactions were when he saw her." Ellen added, "I have watched to see whether he looks over the *Cosmo*-like maga-zines found at the supermarket checkout. He does well!"

It's good for a man to know that his wife is watching from time to time. It helps keep him strong.

PART V

victory with your mind

your mustang mind

As you build the outer defense perimeters, you'll find that the perimeter of the eyes goes up much faster than the perimeter of the mind. Why?

First, the mind is far more crafty than your eyes and more difficult to corral. Second, you really can't rein in the mind effectively until the defense perimeter of the eyes is in place. Knowing this, you shouldn't be discouraged if your mind responds more slowly than your eyes.

The great news is that the defense perimeter of the eyes works *with* you to build the perimeter of the mind. The mind needs an object for its lust, so when the eyes view sexual images, the mind has plenty to dance with. Without those images, the mind has an empty dance card. By starving the eyes, you starve the mind as well. Although this alone is not enough—the mind can still create its own lust objects using memories of movies or pictures you saw years ago or by generating fantasies about old girlfriends or the women with whom you work—at least with your eyes under control you won't be overwhelmed by a continuing flood of fresh lust objects as you struggle to learn to control your mind.

YOUR MIND COMING CLEAN

Currently, your brain moves nimbly to lust and to the little pleasure-high it brings. Your brain's "world-view" has always included lustful thinking. Double entendres, daydreams, and other creative forms of sexual thinking are approved pathways, so your mind feels free to run on these paths to pleasure.

But your mind is orderly, and your world-view colors what comes through it. The mind will allow these impure thoughts only if they "fit" the way you look at the world. As you set up the perimeter of defense for your mind, your brain's world-view will be transformed by a new matrix of allowed thoughts, or "allowables."

Within the old matrix of your thinking, lust fit perfectly and in that sense was "orderly." But with a new, purer matrix firmly in place, lustful thoughts will bring disorder. Your brain, acting as a responsible policeman, nabs these lustful thoughts even before they rise to consciousness. Essentially the brain begins cleaning itself, so elusive enemies like double entendres and daydreams, which are hard to control on the conscious level, simply vanish on their own.

This transformation of the mind takes some time as you wait for the old sexual pollution to be washed away. It's much like living near a creek that becomes polluted when a sewer main breaks upstream. After repair crews replace the cracked sewage pipe, it will still take some time for the water downstream to clear.

In transforming your mind, you'll be taking an active, conscious role in capturing rogue thoughts, but in the long run, the mind will wash itself and will begin to work naturally for you and your purity by capturing such thoughts. With the eyes bouncing away from sexual images and the mind policing itself, your defenses will grow incredibly strong.

LURKING AT THE DOOR

With that confidence, you'll want to be doing all you can to push along your mental transformation.

A helpful concept of something to be on the lookout for is the scriptural imagery of "lurking at the door." Job mentioned it. Just a few verses after we read about the covenant he made with his eyes, we hear Job saying this:

> If my heart has been enticed by a woman,
>   or if I have lurked at my neighbor's door,
> then may my wife grind another man's grain,
>   and may other men sleep with her.
> For that would have been shameful,
>   a sin to be judged. (Job 31:9-11)

Have you "lurked at your neighbor's door"? It could mean stopping by in the late afternoon, visiting your friend's wife for coffee, enamored by her wisdom, care, and sensitivity. You felt sorry for her as you've commiserated together over her insensitive, brutish husband. You held her as she cried. You were lurking at your neighbor's door.

Consider Kevin, who is married with three kids. While working with the youth group at church, he met a beautiful fifteen-year-old girl. "She's a knockout, and looks more like twenty," he said. "Sometimes I'd ask about boys she's known and dated, and we'd joke and laugh a lot, but sometimes I went too far. We'd get to talking a little trashy, about what she liked when kissing, what I bet she wouldn't do with a guy, that sort of thing. I knew I shouldn't talk to her like that, but it was exciting.

"Last week, when my wife and kids were out of town, I gave this girl a ride home. We got to talking dirty again, and somehow I bet her that she wouldn't pull her pants down for me. She did. I lost my senses, and I drove her to a park and we had sex. I'm in real trouble! She told her parents about it, and they may press rape charges!"

Kevin wasn't just lurking at his neighbor's door. Kevin was *inside* his neighbor's door.

Mental Lurking

Maybe you've never done what Kevin did, but you've been lurking at your neighbor's door just the same. According to Jesus, doing it mentally is the same as doing it physically.

You know you've lurked. Your friend's wife seems more like your type than your wife does. *Why didn't I meet her sooner?* you wonder. *How different things would have been if I had.*

Maybe your old girlfriend is married now, yet you lurk at her door in your mind, wondering if she misses you, secretly hoping to run into her at the mall.

Or you've been lunching with a group at work, including that beautiful young sales associate, getting so attached that you're depressed whenever she calls in sick. The last time you sent her an e-mail saying, "I missed you today…hope you feel better soon."

Maybe you've connected with a woman in a chat room, and you imagine what she looks like and what life with her would be like. You're lurking at your neighbor's door.

Wild Thinking

As we've seen, most sexual impurity is generated from women you don't even know. You essentially view them in passing. Models, actresses, receptionists, and pinups are everywhere. But they're strangers. You don't *live* with them, so training the eyes defends against them.

But bouncing your eyes cannot screen out these "live" attractions, attractions from your interactions with women. These women aren't strangers. You live and work in close proximity with them, even worshiping with them on Sundays. Impure thoughts and attractions may arise. Since the defense perimeter of the eyes can't stop them, you need another defense.

"What am I supposed to do?" you say. "Those thoughts come on their own. I can't help them." That certainly *seems* true, since controlling the mind can seem bizarre. Even in church, a daydream may suddenly transpire about some woman at work. Where do these thoughts come from? The mind is like a wild mustang, running free, one thought triggering another in no real order. Still, the Bible says we must control not just our eyes, but our whole bodies:

> You are not your own; you were bought at a price. Therefore
> honor God with your body. (1 Corinthians 6:19-20)

And not just our bodies, but our minds as well. The Holy Spirit, through Paul, is clear on this:

> We demolish arguments and every pretension that sets itself
> up against the knowledge of God, and we take captive every
> thought to make it obedient to Christ. (2 Corinthians 10:5)

This is a jarring verse. Reading it, it's easy to wonder, *Take every thought captive? Is that really possible?*

YOUR MENTAL CUSTOMS STATION

All impure thoughts generate from processing both visual and live attractions through your senses. Viewing women on the beach. Flirting with the new woman at work. Remembering an old girlfriend. During improper processing, our minds can get carried away in impurity. However, by *properly processing* these attractions, we can capture or eliminate impure thoughts.

We've already discussed one form of proper processing called bouncing the eyes. It processes visual attractions by training the eyes to bounce and then starving them. When it's effectively established, your defense perimeter of the eyes has the nature of the old Berlin Wall. No visual entry visas are ever granted for any reason.

But the defense perimeter of the mind is less like a wall and more like a customs area in an international airport. Customs departments are filters, preventing dangerous elements from entering a country. The U.S. Customs Service attempts to filter out drugs, Mediterranean fruit flies, terrorists, and other harmful agents.

Similarly, the defense perimeter of the mind *properly processes* attractive women into your "country," filtering out the alien seeds of attraction before the impure thoughts are even generated. This perimeter "stops the lurking."

Consider the situations of two men we've talked about. Wally, the businessman who dreaded being alone in hotel rooms, found that after turning off the TV, his mind still raced with images in circle after circle of lustful bombardment until he couldn't sleep at all. Had he granted no visual entry visas by watching TV, no lustful thoughts would have been born.

The situation is different for "live" attractions. Kevin was a youth group leader, and that fifteen-year-old girl was a youth group member. She had a valid entry visa into his life. He *had* to interact with her. (Of course, he didn't have to interact improperly.) Attractive women *will* pass through this defense perimeter, but they must only be allowed to enter for appropriate purposes.

FILLING IN THE BLANKS

What happens at our mental customs station?

Say your company hires a new coworker, Rachel. On her first day, Rachel walks around the corner, starts talking, and wham! You're attracted. From this point, she can either be processed properly in your mind without generating impure thoughts, or you can mishandle the situation.

What happens next is critical to the purity of your mind.

You continue interacting with Rachel over time. The early interactions feed the attraction. For instance, Rachel might return your attraction signals. Or her sense of humor may match yours. She loves your favorite pizza. She's simply mad about football. Rachel is refreshing and fascinating, so you love to think about her.

At this point, improper processing carries you away into sensual thoughts or other impure practices, like flirting and teasing. At worst, you can be swept away like the foolish young man in Proverbs 7.

> With persuasive words she led him astray;
> > she seduced him with her smooth talk.
> All at once he followed her
> > like an ox going to the slaughter,
> like a deer stepping into a noose
> > till an arrow pierces his liver,
> like a bird darting into a snare,
> > little knowing it will cost him his life. (7:21-23)

Your mind gets lost in the attractions. It doesn't really matter that you don't know Rachel very well. Early in the relationship, the mind is nimble in filling in the blanks with its creative imagination. That's part of the fun. The less you know about her, the more blanks there are to fill, and the more your mind can run with its fanciful thoughts. With further interaction, however, more facts dribble in. With fewer blanks to fill, the mind quickly gets bored. Facts are the killer virus of attractions.

What kind of facts? Once you've heard her talk about her wonderful new baby and how great her husband is, it becomes harder to imagine Rachel as your "enchantress in waiting." She falls off your attraction screen, becoming merely a friend or coworker.

FROM FRED: LEARNING THE RIGHT
MENTAL PROCESSING

Probably all of us can think of an example from high school where our minds got lost in our attractions. I had one in high school; her name was Judy.

I noticed her early in my senior year, when Judy was a junior. You talk about hitting attraction buttons! I was carried away into a land of silly dreaminess whenever I thought about her. I thought about what I would say and how we would love each other and where we would go, my mind filling in billions of blanks since I knew nothing about Judy except her name and her grade.

All year long I dreamily longed for her, watching her bounce merrily by, hoping for the day we could speak. I yearned to ask her for a date, but I lacked courage. Even though I was the superstud athlete of the year, with girls my heart turned to raspberry Jell-O.

As the year wound down, one chance remained: the senior prom.

Struggling fiercely, I dialed her phone number. After some meaningless small talk, I stammered out my request. She actually said yes! Her melodious voice affirmed my existence, and you can imagine what my mind did with that.

After the prom dance, I found the perfect place to take her—the Ironmen Inn. While the traditional site for after-prom dinners was the Highlander, I decided that I couldn't give my newfound love something so trite and dreary. In the secluded, curtained booths at the Ironmen, we could sit transfixed and not be interrupted on that glorious first night of the rest of our lives together. After being escorted to our booth, we bantered lightly, my heart pounding deeply within me. My attraction grew with each passing moment.

Quietly secluded at the Ironmen, the hostess romantically drew the curtains. Judy's ravishing face glowed, and her lovely, full lips parted to speak. Enchanted, I listened dreamily, only to hear her say, "You know, I don't know how to say this, but I really, really wanted to go to the Highlander. Do you mind if we go over there?"

Clunk.

Although my attraction for her shuddered wildly, chivalry and honor carried the day. Mustering an air of nonchalance, I responded, "Sure, I guess so," though I knew this wasn't good for our date.

At the Highlander, as we stood waiting to be seated, Judy brazenly asked, "Do you mind if I go over to Joel's table for a while?" She left me and spent the rest of the night with him.

I ate alone with my thoughts, musing, *This is why I like football better than girls.*

Later she graciously threw me a bone, allowing me the honor of driving Her Highness home. She confided that she'd hoped all along to find a way to be with Joel that night since he hadn't asked her to the prom as she had expected.

My attractions to Judy died that night. The facts did them in! Initially, I didn't process my attractions to her properly at all. But let me share an example of someone who *did* process some attractions well.

Kirk told me about Patricia, a new woman in his engineering department. When he first saw her, she was giving a presentation to the whole group, and he was hit between the eyes. "I was sitting there expecting another boring presentation when up bops Patricia. She was pretty and intelligent, yet she had an airy disposition. She reminded me so much of the girls I knew back in college. My mind kept insisting, *I've got to get to know this girl, I've got to get to know this girl.* But I was married, and I knew I shouldn't.

"My mind kept demanding to think about her. She seemed so attractive, but I knew I shouldn't think about her. The next few weeks I spent little time around her and didn't talk to her unless I absolutely had to. I starved my eyes from her as well.

"Then I found out she'd just had a baby, and all she could do was talk about her new daughter. She plainly loved her husband very much. At this time, my attractions went down, but not quite out.

"Later, some of the new engineering processes she put into place began to take some heavy criticism, and I saw that her disposition wasn't so light and airy after all. She could be downright shrewish! Today, she's just a friend. I'm not even attracted to her anymore."

STARVING THE ATTRACTIONS

That was proper processing. Patricia had an entry visa, but the attractions were processed properly and generated few impure thoughts. You see, we can't eliminate attractive women from our lives, but we can shield ourselves from the early attraction phase until they become "only friends." This proper processing is called *starving the attractions*.

It's a concept that reminds me of an old cheer from my college days at Stanford:

> *If you can't win, cheat!*
> *If you can't cheat, stall!*
> *If you can't stall, quit!*

Less than admirable, but funny in its way and somewhat applicable here. *Starving the attractions* is a stall tactic. You'll see it in detail later, but active stalling waits for the facts that quickly process the relationship beyond the danger zone, where it generates no impurity.

What happens if we don't starve the attractions? What if we play with the attractions a little? Won't the passage of time kill the attractions anyway?

Most of the time, yes, but you can't take a chance. An improper relationship is not pleasing to God, no matter how "innocent" it appears.

In summary, you have a mind that runs where it wills. It must be tamed. Our best tactic is to starve the attractions, limiting the generation of impure thoughts and the damage they bring to our marriage relationship.

A CORRAL FOR YOUR MUSTANG MIND

We said earlier that our minds are like wild mustangs running free. Mustangs have two characteristics that resemble male brains. First, the mustang runs where he wills. Second, the mustang *mates* where he wills and with whom he chooses. There are mares everywhere! And if a mustang doesn't happen to see one nearby, he'll sniff the wind and, sensing the mare over the horizon, he'll run over there and mate.

This trait is similar to the wild donkey that God talked about through the prophet Jeremiah:

> A wild donkey accustomed to the desert,
> > sniffing the wind in her craving—
> > in her heat who can restrain her?
> Any males that pursue her need not tire themselves;
> > at mating time they will find her. (Jeremiah 2:24)

Can you control the mustang? Can you run him down on foot or simply wag your finger and admonish him? No, of course not. Then how do you keep him from running and mating where he wills?

With a corral.

Currently, your mind runs like a mustang. What's more, your mind "mates" where it wills with attractive, sensual women. They're everywhere.

With a mustang mind, how do you stop the running and the mating? With a corral around your mind.

Let's expand a bit on this metaphor to help you better understand our goal of reining in our roving minds.

Once, you were a proud mustang, wild and free. Sleek and rippling, you ranged the hills and valleys, running and mating where you willed, master of your destiny. God, owner of a large local ranch, noticed you from a distance as He worked His herd. Though you took no notice of Him, He loved you and desired to make you His own. He sought you in many ways, but you ran from Him again and again.

One day He found you trapped in a deep, dark canyon, with no way out. With the lariat of salvation, He gently drew you near, and you became one of His own. He desired to break you, that you might be useful to Him and bring Him further joy. But knowing your natural ways and how you loved to run free with the mares, He set a fence around you. This corral was the perimeter of the eyes. It stopped the running and kept you from sniffing the winds and running wildly over the horizon.

While the corral stopped the running, it hasn't yet stopped the mating. You mate in your mind, through attractions, thoughts, and fantasy, flirting and neighing lustily at the mares inside or near your corral. You must be broken.

Closer and Closer

In light of this picture, let's look at four categories of attractions that have come or will come your way.

The first category is your visual attraction to the strangers we spoke of earlier: the joggers, receptionists, and pinups. Because we've established a defense perimeter of the eyes—our corral—these are now over the horizon. We can't run there anymore. They no longer create attractions.

But there are still plenty of attractions within range of the corral. Categories two through four include the women who are not strangers, the women you interact with in life—the "live" attractions.

In the second category are the women who aren't attractive to you and don't generate impure thoughts. They can include your friends, acquaintances, coworkers, and church members.

Your friend Joe may notice someone and say, "Wow, look at her! She's hot!" You respond in mild surprise, saying, "I guess so. I've worked with her so long I don't even think of her in those terms. She's just a friend."

Your defense against this category of women is a simple monitoring, to make sure you notice early if one of them takes a step toward your corral.

The third category is likely the most dangerous of all. These are the women you know and interact with and who hit your attractions buttons, like Rachel, your new coworker, or maybe the new worship leader who thrills your soul with her keyboard and worshipful heart. You neigh, drawing them toward your corral, if only in your mind.

Perhaps one of them has noticed you as well. Attracted to you, she trots purposefully toward your corral. Flattered, you snort majestically and stomp your foot and toss your head. Looking at her brings much pleasure. Pushing the boundaries, you stretch your head over the fence, nuzzling a bit through private lunches and close conversations. Worst of all, your mustang mind can do something a real mustang could never do—open the gate of the corral. And not just mentally.

Duane told us of a cousin who divorced his wife of twenty-six years after falling head over heels for another woman. "I just didn't know what to say to my cousin," he told us. "He got carried away, and he wasn't going to stop seeing her. There was just no talking to him."

You might say you could never open the gate of your corral to someone in the way Duane's cousin did. But look at statistics for the church, friend. Our divorce rates are no different from the world's. Christians everywhere are separating or recovering from adulterous affairs born of men who opened the corral of their minds. Without defenses, it could happen to you.

The last category includes those women who are already inside your mental corral. Your first thought may be that only your wife is in this category, but there are others whom God has placed close to you. This category can include the wife of your close friend. You'll share restaurant tables with them, create joyful memories with them, and pray earnestly with them. Emotionally, you'll be close. But you must not lurk.

Also inside your corral may be an old girlfriend to whom you're still deeply attached. She was in your corral long before your wife, but she's never been sent out toward the horizon. You mate easily with her in your mind because of your many trysts together. Mentally, she's still right next to you.

Then there's your ex-wife, perhaps the mother of your children. Because of those precious little ones, she'll usually live near you. Because of your former intimacy, she may seem yours for the taking in your mind. You remember the thrills and feel free to play with the thoughts. But you must lead her out of your corral toward the safe horizon.

The perimeter of the mind processes the live attractions that canter up over the horizon and pass our corrals. By starving the attractions, these women retreat to safety zones of "friendship" or "acquaintance," where they no longer threaten our purity. Remember what Kirk said about Patricia? After starving the attractions, she became "just a friend," and he wasn't attracted to her anymore.

Most women won't hit any attraction buttons at all, of course. As they enter your life, they simply trot past your corral toward the horizon. You don't notice them, and they don't notice you. They are and will be merely friends, acquaintances, and coworkers, somewhere off on the horizon. But those who *do* attract you and *do* approach your corral must not be given any reason to come closer or even approach the gate, where you just might, in a moment of weakness, let her in.

PREVENTING SAD STORIES

Don't you owe it to your wife to put up a mental defense perimeter? You *must* protect your wife and kids from attractions outside your corral; otherwise, you'll have a sad story to tell, like the one we heard from Jack.

Jack was involved in full-time Christian ministry, standing strong. He had no mental defense perimeter, however, because he blissfully thought he didn't need one. As a result he allowed Mary to come too close to his corral.

"Mary attended my church and was involved in the music ministry," Jack told us. "Because of my skills and position in the church, I was involved in many activities with her. We were in a small worship band, and during practices I noticed she began smiling in that certain way. She was pretty, and I was attracted, but I didn't give it much thought until she kept smiling at me. I got to thinking about it. The attractions were growing, and I felt a little excited and pleased with myself.

"One day, she stopped by my office and caught me alone. She began pouring out her troubles with her husband. As a minister, I often did counseling, so I felt I should listen. She started crying, and I put my arms around her, feeling sorry for her. She snuggled in a little, and I kind of liked it. She left, and nothing came of it, but now I was thinking about her constantly.

"Mary and I happened to take the same road to work, and I noticed she would be watching for me each morning, waving and smiling. At practice, she was more and more flattering of my musical talents. She looked at me with those eyes even when I preached, smiling slightly, though sitting right next to her husband. It was kind of naughty and thrilling.

"I began doing the strangest things, like driving miles out of my way to her office, just to see her car. What in the world did I gain by seeing her car, for Pete's sake? But it was romantic somehow. Finally, a few weeks later we were alone, and I kissed her. I knew that kiss would end my career at my church, but I couldn't help myself. The attraction had grown too strong."

Jack's career, marriage, and relationships with his children were severely damaged that afternoon. He said it could never happen, but it did happen because Jack lacked a defense perimeter.

Your wife and kids deserve a defense, friend. You never know who will gallop near your corral.

approaching your corral

Here's another helpful way of analyzing the "live" attractions in your life and what they mean for your mental defense perimeter.

Let's think about two types of women who will approach your corral:

- Women you find attractive
- Women who find you attractive

Both categories have similar defenses, each designed to starve the attractions until she trots off toward the horizon. Here's a closer look.

WOMEN YOU FIND ATTRACTIVE

If you find someone attractive, your first line of defense is a proper mind-set, which is this: *This attraction threatens everything I hold dear.*

It may not appear threatening early in the attraction, when everything seems innocent. Remember, though, that attractions grow quickly and can destroy your marriage. Even if your marriage manages to survive, at the very least the lurking will weaken the foundation of your marriage and rob your wife of your full captivation.

Your second line of defense is to declare, *I have no right to think these things.* State this to yourself clearly, decisively, and often. You don't even *know* this woman; who are you to be attracted to her? Didn't your Master give you *your* wife?

The third line of defense is to heighten your alert. What do you normally do when you feel threatened? You take off your jacket and breathe deeply. You ready yourself for what's coming.

Suppose you are a bouncer at a dance club, checking I.D.s and tickets, joking with the customers. One night, five men in black leather loudly roar up on motorcycles, looking surly and arrogant. Would you relax and back away from the door? Not on your life. Without hesitation, you'd step up to the door and stand erect, ready to confront the threat.

Consider the old *Star Trek* television series. What did Captain Kirk do when danger approached? He cried out: "Red alert! Shields up!" In a similar vein, when an attractive woman approaches your corral, your defense perimeter must immediately respond: *Red alert! Shields up!*

With your mind-set transformed, you won't let her near the corral. The attraction will begin to starve, and she'll drift back toward the horizon.

How can you make sure that will happen?

Bounce your eyes. You *saw* her passing your corral, and you were *physically* attracted to her. Starve this attraction by bouncing your eyes. Don't dwell on her beauty by stealing glances. Do this with zeal.

Avoid her. Sometimes this isn't possible, but do it when you can. If she works with you, and the two of you are assigned to the same project, don't ask her to eat lunch with you or offer her a ride home. Avoid opportunities that create positive experiences with her until the attraction phase dies. If she asks you to do something with her, excuse yourself.

When you're in her company, play the dweeb. Our hero, Dweebman, steps into a nearby public rest room and emerges as the polyester-clad enemy of all things flirtatious and hip. Dull, mild-mannered Dweebman—pocket protector shielding his heart and hair slightly askew—wages his quiet, thankless war of boring interchange. Our once-threatening Amazon withdraws to undefended sectors, leaving Dweebman victorious again in his never-ending good fight to stave off the hip and the impure in his galactic empire!

Okay, there's not *that* much glory in playing the dweeb. There'll be no comic-book deals, no endorsement deals, no *20/20* interviews with Barbara Walters, but you'll be a hero to your wife and kids.

A dweeb is the opposite of a *player*. In relationships, players send and receive social signals smoothly. Dweebs do not. When a player wants to send attraction signals, there are certain things he'll do. He'll flirt. He'll banter. He'll smile with a knowing look. He'll talk about hip things. In short, he'll be cool. You were a player at one time. You knew how to feed attractions. You spent your whole adolescence learning how.

As a married man, however, a little social suicide is very much in order. *Always* play the dweeb. Players flirt…learn to un-flirt. Players banter… learn to un-banter. If a woman smiles with a knowing look, learn to smile with a slightly confused look, to un-smile. If she talks about things that are hip, talk about things that are un-hip to her, like your wife and kids. She'll find you pleasant enough but rather bland and uninteresting. Perfect.

Sometimes a woman's attractiveness to you will be mental rather than physical. This is common in work environments as you work with women on projects that interest you both. In business it's common to spend more hours per day with female coworkers than with your wife. You talk with them about common goals and achieving success, while all you and your wife talk about are the kids' discipline problems, who's going to change the dirty diapers, and bills, bills, bills.

As with physically attractive women, you must understand that if your shields aren't up, and if you don't recognize the threat to your marriage, you're flirting with danger.

To summarize: If you're attracted to a woman, it doesn't mean you may never again have any sort of relationship or friendship with her. It only means you must enact your defense perimeters. Once you've starved the attractions and she's a safe distance away, you can have a proper relationship, one that is honoring to your wife and to the Lord.

WOMEN WHO FIND YOU ATTRACTIVE

No matter what our age (or our waistlines), we're still capable of saying preposterous things like, "Finally, *here* is a woman who clearly has good taste and knows 'handsome' when she sees it. I simply *must* get to know her better." Yes, guys still make those statements.

Ed, being short on cash, took a second job working an early shift at FedEx to make ends meet. He was simply doing what a man should do for his family during a serious financial crunch. When Christi, an aggressive, attractive dispatcher, pranced by Ed's corral, she said, "You're so cute and sexy! I love to wrap my legs around men like you!" She bantered and flirted at every turn, teasing with double entendres and come-ons. She spread her legs slightly whenever they talked, and her shirt often flopped open for him.

One day she said, "My husband is out of town hunting for the weekend. I'm going to be *so* lonely." *Red alert! Red alert!* An hour later, Ed found her house key on his desk with a note, saying, "I've left you this key in case you need to get into my house this weekend!"

Ed, to his credit, returned her key and let it be known in no uncertain terms that he would not be coming, and he asked her to stop what she was doing. Ed kept the gate to his corral closed, because Christi was threatening everything he held dear.

If a gang of ravenous teens were outside your home, approaching with axes and clubs, you would probably sense a threat. *Red alert! Shields up!* Just as dangerous is the woman who finds you attractive. You must stop her by returning no attraction signals. If she's a non-Christian, she's even more dangerous since she has no moral reason not to go to bed with you.

Your second line of defense is using your shield of rights. *I have no right to think these thoughts, and I have no right to return these signals!* Jesus died a bloody death on the cross to purchase you. He has all the rights here. You have none. Speak this out loudly to yourself again and again; it breaks and reins in the mustang mind.

Don't dawdle about getting your shields up. In one *Star Trek* movie episode, the enemy had captured a Federation starship and was approaching Kirk and the starship *Enterprise* (the good guys). The enemy commander didn't respond to any calls from Kirk. As Kirk hailed him repeatedly, the enemy commander simply sneered, "Let them eat static."

Kirk found this lack of response peculiar. Confused and unsure of the intentions of the approaching ship, he dawdled. He did not put up his shields. Finally, when close enough, the enemy blasted away, severely disabling the *Enterprise*. Kirk paid a dear price for dawdling, losing his best friend to death in the ensuing interchanges.

When a woman approaches your corral, you don't know what her intentions are. Maybe you're misreading her bright, outgoing personality, and she isn't attracted to you at all. Maybe she greets everyone that way. Maybe not. There may be an enemy on that ship. Get your shields up and ask questions later. Don't pay that dear price.

What do you do when someone finds you attractive? How do you starve these attractions? Here are some guidelines:

Spend absolutely no time alone with this woman, even in public places. The reason is simple. You don't want to feed her attractions. Make it obvious you aren't returning her interest in you.

Flee from her. Don't smile knowingly at her. Don't join her prayer group. Don't join her worship team. Avoid working with her on a committee. Don't be anywhere that she can be further impressed with you. Do this consciously and methodically.

Prepare with "war game" simulations. What will you say if she calls you at work? What will you do if she invites you to lunch? Josh McDowell tells teens to decide what they'll do in the backseat of the car *before* they ever get to the backseat of the car. Otherwise passion rules, and reasoning isn't clear.

As adults, we applaud his advice to teenagers. Why not follow Josh's words ourselves?

Send absolutely no return attraction signals. Don't answer the call. *Let them eat static!*

Play the dweeb. Help her out. Show her that her initial attraction to you was a ridiculous mistake. Choose to be boring, and do it fastidiously. Later, when she's no longer attracted to you, you can be your normal, interesting self again.

inside your corral

For those women who are already within your corral, the situation becomes rather complicated. These women won't drift back to the horizon. They're in your corral today and probably will be there tomorrow and the next day. This means you must eliminate these attractions in some other way.

Let's take a look at the two main categories of women within your corral.

- Old girlfriends and ex-wives
- Wives of your friends

Again, not every woman in these categories will be attractive to you. But if one of these women catches your fancy or has retained a piece of your heart, something must be done. Each category has unique dangers, and each demands unique defenses, so let's take a look at what we should do.

FROM FRED: OLD FLAME

An old girlfriend or an ex-wife can be deadly to mental purity. Such attractions break you down in two ways:

- They weaken your ability to move toward one flesh with your wife.
- They enable Satan to fire a cruise missile, with little warning, into your marriage.

I had a heart-stopping summer romance with Polly following my freshman year of college. At the end of the summer, I left her to return to school in California. Lonely and heartsick, I wandered aimlessly through my days, feeling sorry for myself. We wrote every day and telephoned often. This went on for much of the fall quarter.

One day during an intramural football game, my eyes caught sight of a female referee. She looked like a grown-up version of my childhood sweetheart, Melody Knight, who had moved to Canada when we were in the third grade.

After the game, I walked up and asked her what her name was (that was the extent of my "lines" in those days). Had she said, "Melody," I'd have instantly fallen for her. Instead, she said her name was Betsy, and I fell for her instantly anyway. (As you can see, if anyone ever needed good defenses, it was me!)

My attraction to Betsy played itself out fairly soon. Meanwhile, Polly wondered why the letters and phone calls stopped. When I finally got the nerve to tell her there was someone else in my life, she was hurt deeply. When my little relationship with Betsy ended, I asked Polly for mercy and a second chance, but she would have none of it. Loyalty meant everything to her, and my breach of loyalty killed any attraction she felt for me.

But I was no quitter. I fought on, longing for her for many years. Whenever I had a new girlfriend and things turned stormy, I dreamed of Polly, wishing she were mine. "Everything would be different with Polly," I'd moan.

Polly eventually married and had two children. But I was still so hooked that after a separation from her husband, I begged for her love again. (This was before I met Brenda, of course.) "Kids, debts, baggage—I'll carry them all, just to have you back," I begged. You could have made a syrupy movie about my puppy love for Polly.

With such an image of "undying" love for Polly, it's no wonder that when I finally fell in love with Brenda and married her, I didn't know what was coming. A tranquil tunnel of love? More like a roller coaster!

Brenda and I have had our share of fights, starting just days after the honeymoon. In fact, at times during our first two years of marriage I wished I had never heard of the institution. Most of our conflicts were over in-laws, especially after my family engaged my new bride in a war, and I got caught in the middle. The fights were hot and withering. Being young, we didn't know how to fight fair with each other or with our family members, so the collateral damage was great; we both suffered major losses.

Guess who popped into my thought life? As my marriage spiraled downward, Polly spiraled upward into my thoughts. *Well, Polly always got along with my family. They loved her.* Around the holidays, I mused how peaceful life would have been with Polly. *Why can't Brenda get along with my family? After all, Polly could!*

No Right

One night I was driving on an Iowa road between Fort Dodge and Harcourt. The moon was full, and the air was crisp and clear. As Polly popped into my head, an insight popped in as well, and I said to myself, *You have no right to any relationship of any type with Polly anymore, even in your thoughts.*

What? No right to even *think* about her?

That's right, buddy. No right to even think of her.

How stark! My mind rebelled fiercely, and the fight was on. My mind *liked* Polly, and it *fought* for her. In the end, however, truth prevailed. I knew I'd forsaken all others on my wedding day. This promise had to become true in practice and not just in words.

Polly had been a girlfriend and had long been inside my corral, but it was time for me to open the gate and show her out. She had a husband whose hopes and dreams were tied up in her, and she had children who loved her. I had no right to my thoughts, even if Polly knew nothing (and she didn't). Besides, Brenda deserved better from me.

I needed to capture my thoughts about Polly and obliterate my attraction to her. I found the process far simpler than I thought it would be. I obliterated all "memory anchors," destroying every old card, letter, and picture of her. All traces of Polly were eliminated, just as God's people were supposed to do with the Canaanites when they entered the Promised Land.

These actions improved the situation, but Polly's anchors weren't the only issue. I had to destroy my memories of her as well, because they stood in opposition to God's desires and hopes for my marriage.

How do I do that? I wondered. I wasn't sure, but I had to try.

First, I prayed for understanding and insight since I didn't know what I was doing. Then I stumbled ahead as best I knew how. I began by using the shield of rights every time Polly entered my head. I coldly stated, *I have no right to think about Polly, and I won't.*

Having said that, I would sing a hymn or quote a Scripture. Why? In the early days, I found that if I cast out a thought, a void remained. Without filling the void, "Polly thoughts" rushed back in. So I sang softly to fill the voids. It was a tough battle at first. As a hymn ended, Polly might immediately return, so sometimes it took numerous verses. In due time, I'd always win the skirmish, but within a few hours or a few days the thoughts returned, and I'd fight again.

During those days, I remember thinking, *I cannot take chances by simply detaining these captive thoughts in a detention center. I must nuke these thoughts!* That was a bit corny, but I knew there must be no question of victory when this battle was over.

Over time I began winning decisively. With practice, I could actually grab an incoming impure thought and toss it out without singing, without filling the void. I could *will it* to be gone, and it would go. After yet more time, thoughts of Polly stopped entirely. My brain finally understood that "Polly thoughts" were unapproved.

SATAN'S CRUISE MISSILES

As mentioned earlier, however, there's a second danger in not taking care of business with the attractions inside the corral. If you're careless, Satan can fire a cruise missile into your marriage and shatter your world in a moment.

Years ago, I noticed a problem with Don, a married friend. He hadn't told me so, but several times when I was at his home, I noticed his finger hesitate on the TV remote when passing sex scenes on the movie channels. While the hesitation was nearly imperceptible, I saw it easily. His eyes had no defense, so I knew what he'd been watching. What I didn't know, until it was too late, was what he'd also been *thinking*.

Don and his wife were having problems. To him, the worst were the sexual frustrations. "Joann just doesn't fulfill me," he told me. "It wouldn't take much because I don't ask for much. All I wanted was to French kiss with her. She just wouldn't do it. We'd be messing around and, as things heated up, I'd try some French kissing. She always got angry and pulled away. She says it's filthy and makes her nauseous. I don't see how French kissing is any filthier than any other kiss. It's the same saliva! Besides the Bible says that her body is not her own, but it's actually mine. The Bible gives me a right to sexual fulfillment, and as my wife, she *owes* me sexual fulfillment. It wasn't fair, and I didn't know what to do."

Actually, Don had already decided on what to do and that was to turn his thoughts to his old girlfriend, where he could daydream about her French kisses and what might have been. She *loved* French kissing. Don was ripe for the taking.

He hadn't heard from this old flame in years, and he figured his thoughts were harmless. What could they hurt? He didn't even know where she was, but Satan did. Out of the blue, she called Don and said she'd be in town. Don's unguarded mind raced with the possibilities at a time when his defense perimeters were down.

The two of them landed in a hotel room. Boom! He didn't think it could happen to him, but in one smashing blow, his marriage was blasted to smithereens. He couldn't say no.

Bottom line: You have *no right* to any relationship with an old girl-friend or ex-wife if you still nurture an attraction to her.

FRIENDS' WIVES

You may think affairs like Don's happen so infrequently that you can confidently say, "Well, *I* would never do such a thing!" But words like that mean nothing if you have any sense. We urge you: Please, protect yourself. Don't be defenseless because you *can* get fooled.

Far too much is at stake to be sloppy with your defenses with anyone, and that includes the wives of your friends. If your best friend gave you all his worldly goods and told you to take care of them, you would probably invest wisely and take no chances. More important, you should take no chances with his wife, his most precious love of all.

Have you ever had an attraction to a friend's wife at any time? Without defense perimeters, you've probably had many attractions. You're a man. Attractions happen. What do you do?

Again, you start with the truth: *I have no right to any relationship with my friend's wife apart from my relationship with my friend.* Remember especially that there's nothing more dangerous than talking to a friend's wife when things are dry in either your marriage or her marriage.

It's not that you don't trust your friend's wife; it's that you don't want to start anything. She should be like a sister to you, with no hint of attraction between you.

You'll always have *some* relationship with your friend's wife, but limit it to when your friend is around. This isn't always possible, but these simple rules can shield you from surprise attacks within the corral:

1. Limit all conversations between you and your friend's spouse unless your wife or your friend is with you. Keep things light and short, like vanilla.

2. If you phone your friend and he isn't home, get off the line with his wife promptly. Don't be rude, but don't plan on talking more than briefly with her.

3. If you stop by your friend's house and he isn't home, she may invite you in. What do you do then? Politely decline to enter. What possible purpose is served by staying?

4. Capture any attractions toward your friend's wife and nuke them totally. Return to the rules of starving the eyes and taking such thoughts captive. Never, ever tell yourself, "Oh, I can handle it— no problem." You need to deliberately tear away the thoughts so she doesn't see the attraction signals and decide to send back a few of her own. Leave her no opportunity to send a return signal.

You may view these precautions as overly strict and tight, but we're counseling safety measures. In practice, this approach isn't restrictive. Your friends' wives are with your friends most of the time, so the rules don't apply that often. You're rarely alone with a friend's spouse.

What God has put together, let no man tear asunder. Protect your friend's hopes and dreams as diligently as you're protecting your *own* hopes and dreams. You're his friend. Given the divorce statistics within the church, a simple defense perimeter isn't too much to ask of yourself.

And some advice for a special situation: If you're single and a close female friend gets married, be willing to quickly and graciously let the friendship drift away. Marriage changes things. She's no longer the same person. Mysteriously, she is now one flesh with another man. She needs to be about building her marital relationship and finding "couple friends" together with him.

FROM FRED: LEARNING A LESSON

Before I knew Brenda, my best friend was a woman named Terry who lived in the apartment above me. She had a boyfriend to whom she was perfectly loyal, and I wasn't in the market for a girlfriend at the time, so we paired well. We would often sit for hours as she talked about her insecurities, fears, and frustrations. I had just moved back to Iowa from California, and she was the only close friend I had.

Then I met Brenda, whom I courted mostly by phone during our seven-month romance. Since she lived in another city three hours away, Brenda had little to do with Terry. Shortly after we were married, I told Brenda that I was planning to have lunch with Terry the following Wednesday.

"Why?" Brenda asked.

"To catch up on things mostly."

"And I'm not invited?"

"Well, she's having some personal problems she wants to talk over with me, and since you don't know each other, she would probably feel uncomfortable sharing them in front of you."

"I'm not sure I like that."

"Why?" I asked. "We've always been just friends."

"Well, for one thing," she explained, "I'm not sure I'm comfortable with us having friends of the opposite sex without each other. Besides, it looks bad for you to have lunch with a single woman alone. What if someone from church saw you? I just don't feel right about it."

"You trust me, don't you?"

"I trust you. And she has a boyfriend, so I trust her motives for now. But what if her motives change down the line? I won't be there to spot it."

I pondered Brenda's reasoning and eventually canceled the lunch date. It made sense. I'd learned that it wasn't appropriate for me to have lunch with Terry.

I was glad I listened to Brenda's advice. As my own marriage struggled during the first two years, I was glad I only had to deal with the memories of Polly. Had Terry been around, who knows what would have happened? Though we were never romantically involved, our closeness and intimacy might have turned romantic. As a new Christian, would I have been able to resist falling for her? Given my track record, I'm glad Brenda dismissed that friendship early on.

Some would say that all such friendships with the opposite sex should die once one marries. While I wouldn't go that far, I *will* say that such friendships must be guarded. To be careful is to be wise.

SACRIFICE AND BLESSING

In *The Final Quest,* Rick Joyner writes, "Spiritual maturity is always dictated by our willingness to sacrifice our own desires for the desires of others or for the interests of the kingdom."

Purifying your eyes and mind is more than a command—it's also a sacrifice. And as you make that sacrifice, as you lay down your desires, blessings will flow. Your spiritual life will experience new joy and power, and your marriage life will blossom as your relationship reaches new heights.

Experiencing that relationship with all your heart is what the final part of this book will be about.

The Heart of a Woman

Brenda hated this section. "Men seem like untrustworthy pigs whose minds and thoughts just go wherever they want," she commented. "Is *nothing* sacred to them? As women, do we trust men after reading this? You can't even trust a pastor to be a pure person. I feel that if anything ever happened to Fred, I'd never remarry because I would have very little trust in men."

Brenda also thought Fred presented himself as an untrustworthy man in this chapter, especially while talking about Polly and Terry. She said men may not read it that way, but women will.

We won't deny her comments because Fred was untrustworthy. How could he help it? For men, attractions seem to just happen. It's part of being male. Of course, women can also be attracted to other men; it just doesn't happen as often as men being attracted to women.

Brenda said, "I rarely ever pay much attention to other men. I might notice a good-looking guy, but I never give it more than a passing thought. Before marriage I used to worry whether I would ever be attracted to someone else. For some reason that has never come close to happening. I suppose it could happen to women who have unfaithful husbands or whose husbands are lazy toads or insensitive couch potatoes."

Deena agreed. "I *really* have trouble understanding this. As a woman, I don't have this problem."

Cathy, on the other hand, gave a slight concession: "When I see a physically attractive man, I may look and appreciate, but I don't dwell. I've learned to get past the infatuation stage and figure that he's someone who probably has bad breath, picks his nose, and sleeps around on his wife. Even if he doesn't, I have no right to fantasize about this person."

Some men seem to have little problem in this area. Both Andrea and Heather said that though their husbands have had problems with their eyes, they were sure their husbands didn't face this particular problem with their minds.

Of course, most attractions facing men are not sudden, and the slower-forming attractions are the most dangerous. Even women without attraction buttons are subject to these slow-forming attractions, and they must be prepared too. The statistics on adultery are stunning, and both sexes need to understand how dangerous attractions can be.

PART VI

victory in your heart

cherishing your one and only

Your outer defense perimeters—protecting your eyes and your mind—will defend against sexual impurities, guaranteeing that your wife remains beyond compare in your eyes.

Now let's talk about a third perimeter, your innermost perimeter, which is about being consumed with God's purpose to cherish your wife.

WHERE YOUR COMMITMENT TO GOD SHOWS FIRST

If Christians were consumed by God's purposes, it would first be reflected in our marriages. But the rates of divorce, adultery, and marital dissatisfaction in the Christian church reveal our hearts.

We've known very few men consumed by their marriages, and fewer still consumed by purity, but both are God's desire for you. God's purpose for your marriage is that it parallels Christ's relationship to His church, that you be one with your wife.

But what does the standard of Christ's relationship to His church have to do with our sexual purity? In our hearts, we often have selfish attitudes and expectations regarding our wives. When these expectations aren't met, we become grumpy and frustrated. Our will to maintain our outer defense perimeters is eroded. *Well, if this is how she's going to be, why should I go through all the effort of being pure? She doesn't deserve it.* We retaliate by withdrawing from our own responsibilities, but cherishing our wives includes being sexually pure. If this inner defense fails, the outer perimeters of the eyes and mind can also fail—and quite quickly.

Perhaps you're finding it difficult to cherish your one and only. We understand that sentiment. To cherish means to treat with tenderness and to hold dear, and you want to feel the romantic urge to do those things. But what if you don't feel like it? Something with such ramifications upon your sexual purity and upon the very strength of your marriage cannot be left to feelings alone.

How Cherishing Feels

Just how does cherishing feel? Does your wife feel cherished? For centuries the Song of Solomon has often been viewed as an allegory of how Christ feels for His bride and how she feels in return. Keep that interpretation in mind as you read the portions below (condensed from chapters 4–7).

Look first at Jesus' feelings toward His bride:

> *How beautiful you are, my darling!*
> > *Oh, how beautiful!*
> > *Your eyes behind your veil are doves....*
> *Your lips are like a scarlet ribbon;*
> > *Your mouth is lovely....*
> *All beautiful you are, my darling;*
> > *there is no flaw in you....*
> *You have stolen my heart, my sister, my bride;*
> > *you have stolen my heart*
> > *with one glance of your eyes....*

How delightful is your love, my sister, my bride!…
Your head crowns you like Mount Carmel.
   Your hair is like royal tapestry;
   the king is held captive by its tresses.
How beautiful you are and how pleasing,
   O love, with your delights.
      (Song of Songs 4:1,3,7,9-10; 7:5-6)

Now observe the church's feelings toward Jesus:

My lover [husband] is radiant and ruddy,
   outstanding among ten thousand.
His head is purest gold;
   his hair is wavy
   and black as a raven.…
His mouth is sweetness itself;
   he is altogether lovely.
This is my lover, this is my friend.
I belong to my lover,
   and his desire is for me.…
Let us go early to the vineyards…
   there I will give you my love.
The mandrakes send out their fragrance,
   and at our door is every delicacy,
both new and old,
   that I have stored up for you, my lover.
      (Song of Songs 5:10-11,16; 7:10,12-13)

Do you sense Jesus' desire for you as part of His Bride? In return, does your heart yearn for Him like this?

Because our marriage relationships should parallel Christ's relationship to the church, our feelings for our wives should parallel these passages.

What a great reminder of how exciting love can be, especially when channeled toward the one God intended for us to have.

FROM FRED: CAUGHT UP IN CONDITIONS

Do you feel these things for your wife? I haven't always.

Do you remember pop quizzes from school, a sort of diabolical truth serum used by evil teachers to expose your knowledge (or lack of it) to the world? God loves pop quizzes, but He doesn't test our *knowledge* with them. He tests our character.

I'm reminded of that when I recall the times during our first two years of marriage when Brenda and I were staggered by in-law problems with my family. Our marriage was quickly wilting away.

One Valentine's Day, I went to buy a card. Without warning, this turned into a pop quiz from God. Fingering through the cards, I read the texts. One by one I returned them to the rack as "too mushy," "too contrived," or "too romantic." Little by little, panic settled in as I sensed the inevitable. Not one Valentine's card in the store could be sent by me with any measure of sincerity.

Head down, I scurried from the store, recognizing the depth of our loss. My grade on the quiz? Sickening!

What about you? Are you cherishing your wife? Do you feel cherished?

If not, you probably got there the same way I did—by stopping short of God's standards. God's standard is to unconditionally cherish her, no matter what. *No* conditions. But in America, we've added mealy-mouthed terms to form "conditional contracts."

If I were living according to God's purposes, I'd have added no conditions. But in my marriage, my conditions were that I would cherish Brenda *if* she made peace with my family and shaped up.

When we set conditions, we fix our gaze on what we expect to get from the marriage. There's nothing wrong with expecting something, of course, and in premarriage classes, I always ask the question, *What do you expect to get out of marriage that you can't get by staying single?* We hope for an Eden, where needs are met and dreams are fulfilled.

The problem comes when we expect our wives to deliver these things under contractual conditions. With Brenda, anger and resentment erupted when I felt she didn't carry her side of the bargain. I no longer felt like cherishing her.

With that kind of focus, oneness in a marriage can't grow. For instance, Bill said this about his wife: "She was showing such a lack of ambition. What I expected when we got married was that we would both continue in our careers and really build our lives financially in our early years. She just isn't doing what I thought she'd do, and she really seems kind of lazy and selfish. Then she got pregnant. After a few months she said, 'I don't like the way I look anymore, so I don't want to have sex until after the baby comes.' I found that so unfair.

"The thought of no sex bothered me the more I thought about it, and I thought that if she were just going to live any way she pleased, I would live any way I pleased. I have a biblical right to sexual fulfillment, and I'll have it one way or another. That's how I came to have an affair." That's a flimsy excuse for adultery, but its seeds were in Bill's focus on what he wanted out of the marriage.

These kind of conditional contracts don't work because they're written as we go along. Regardless of how long we date, we don't really know each other well enough to cover the hidden or changing conditions of the heart and mind.

For instance, how could I have anticipated the huge problems with my family, and how could Brenda have anticipated my out-of-control temper? I broke holes in walls with my bare hands. I threw pots of bean soup across the kitchen floor. How could she have expected any of this?

A conditional marriage contract originally defines what we hope to get out of marriage. As time passes and we learn more, we add more expectations and more requirements until we hardly recognize the agreement anymore. *Wait a minute! This isn't working out like I expected. I'm getting out!*

Brenda and I came to a moment of truth sometime after that bean soup hit the floor. She simply said, "I don't know how else to say this. My feelings for you are dead." She wondered if we should consider divorce.

Hearing that word stunned me. As a child of divorce, the old feelings of horror swept over me again.

No Matter How Much Gravel

Several days passed. One day when Brenda was at work, I stood before my refrigerator and reached in for a half-gallon of milk. Her words lay heavily upon my chest. I poured the milk, shut the refrigerator door, and paused.

I had to do something.

Raising my right hand and pointing a finger toward heaven, I declared, "God, I don't care how much gravel I have to eat, I'll *never* get a divorce."

I finally understood the promise I'd made on my wedding day. My promise wasn't conditional. If she fed me meat and potatoes, I would eat it. If she fed me gravel, I would eat it. I was going to change or tolerate or love in whatever way necessary, but I would keep my promise to love and cherish her, whatever the cost.

"What does eating gravel have to do with cherishing?" you might ask. "Do I give up everything I have to keep peace? What about *my* rights?"

Well, you do have a few rights, and we're not saying your wife has no responsibility in return. But in the countless ways we poke each other in this shared space called marriage, our focus needs to be on *our* sharp edges, not hers.

God always knew marriages would wither when rooted in contracts, which is why He established unconditional covenants. He knew that conditions change.

God never forgot what we often forget—namely, the curse of Eden is a grinding curse. Life is a steamroller, making pancakes of conditions and easily mashing the naive contracts we create. In our dreams for marriage, maybe we forget that we would still have to work long hours by the sweat of our brow to eat, and that we wouldn't always see each other as much as we wish. Maybe we forget that we will sometimes be beaten up and used by bosses, our minds so numb we just don't want to talk when we get home. Maybe we forget that with the pain in childbirth comes bodies that never regain their former shape.

Any number of trials and tribulations might make conditions impossible to meet, but we demanded guarantees anyway, demanding some form of Eden from our marriages, when all the time our place is to cherish our wives unconditionally.

That doesn't sound much like Eden to us. We don't like our place. So our inner defenses are let down, and we lose our concern for God's purposes.

A MAN WITH COMPLETE FAITHFULNESS

We want to direct your attention now to a man in the Bible who liked his place and loved God's purposes. All men should be as faithful as he was, cherishing both their King and their wives.

This man's name was Uriah.

In 1 Chronicles 11 we see Uriah listed as one of David's "mighty men"—the men who "gave his kingship strong support to extend it over the whole land, as the LORD had promised" (11:10).

Uriah was clearly consumed with the purposes of his king, David. He was also consumed with the purposes of God. Uriah was by David's side in the caves when Saul hounded their heels. He cried with David as their homes burned at Ziklag. He cheered himself hoarse at David's coronation, and he fearlessly fought to extend David's kingdom over the whole land. Swearing his life to the purposes of God, Uriah stood in harm's way for David's throne.

Sound familiar? You swore your life to someone, didn't you? You swore before family and friends to honor and cherish your wife, abandoning all others. You promised she would have more from marriage than she would have as a single woman. Are you consumed by this commitment? Consumed enough to live faithfully and to cherish her completely? Consumed enough to stand in harm's way and to eat gravel until God's purposes and your promises are finally established in your land?

Uriah was that consumed. His faithfulness was complete, but alas, David's faithfulness wasn't. He went to bed with Bathsheba, Uriah's wife. When she became pregnant, he had a mess on his hands. As always, Uriah was out fighting David's battles. Bathsheba's pregnancy could mean only one thing: David—not Uriah—was the father.

David addressed the situation by fabricating a ruse. He ordered Uriah back from the front lines. David's plan was to send Uriah quickly home to a warm, cuddly night with Bathsheba. If David moved quickly enough, people would naturally assume the unborn child was Uriah's.

Tragically, Uriah's faithfulness to the king was so complete that David's plan didn't work:

> David said to Uriah, "Go down to your house and wash
> your feet." So Uriah left the palace, and a gift from the

king was sent after him. But Uriah slept at the entrance
to the palace with all his master's servants and did not
go down to his house.

When David was told, "Uriah did not go home," he
asked him, "Haven't you just come from a distance? Why
didn't you go home?"

Uriah said to David, "The ark and Israel and Judah are
staying in tents, and my master Joab and my lord's men are
camped in the open fields. How could I go to my house to
eat and drink and lie with my wife? As surely as you live, I
will not do such a thing!"

Then David said to him, "Stay here one more day,
and tomorrow I will send you back." So Uriah remained
in Jerusalem that day and the next. At David's invitation,
he ate and drank with him, and David made him drunk.
But in the evening Uriah went out to sleep on his mat
among his master's servants; he did not go home.
(2 Samuel 11:8-13)

Look at Uriah! He was so consumed by the purposes of God that he
refused to go to his house even to wash his feet. His faithfulness was so
strong that, even when drunk, he didn't waver from his commitment and
zeal. His purity of soul was so great that no treacherous trick formed against
him could stand. God wouldn't allow David's simple deception to cover his
great sin against God and against God's choice servant Uriah. God loved
Uriah, and God loved Uriah's love for Bathsheba.

Uriah knew his place. He was satisfied to be part of God's purposes, to
fill his role.

To be like Uriah, we must know our place and be content with it.

Your Ewe Lamb

What does it mean to cherish? We needn't look further than Uriah's example, because his cherishing heart toward Bathsheba was transforming.

After David arranged for Uriah to be killed in battle, God sent His prophet Nathan to confront David with his sin. He used a word-picture story that revealed Uriah's cherishing, loving heart toward Bathsheba:

> The LORD sent Nathan to David. When he came to him, he said, "There were two men in a certain town, one rich and the other poor. The rich man had a very large number of sheep and cattle, but the poor man had nothing except one little ewe lamb he had bought. He raised it, and it grew up with him and his children. It shared his food, drank from his cup and even slept in his arms. It was like a daughter to him.
>
> Now a traveler came to the rich man, but the rich man refrained from taking one of his own sheep or cattle to prepare a meal for the traveler who had come to him. Instead, he took the ewe lamb that belonged to the poor man and prepared it for the one who had come to him." (2 Samuel 12:1-4)

The rich man in the story represented David, who saw Bathsheba only as someone he could devour to satisfy his sexual longings, but Uriah, "the poor man," saw his "lamb" as the joy of his life, his pet to cherish, to sleep in his arms. Uriah had only one wife; a faithful man like him could have only one. His ewe lamb, Bathsheba, bounced and pranced and frolicked and laughed with him, bringing him great joy.

The lamb "was like a daughter to him," the passage says. Do you have daughters? If so, you know what the Lord conveys here. A love for a daughter is special, and daughters are easy to cherish. They speak of Beanie Babies or Barbies or some girl at school with lice in her hair or some boy who spits in the schoolyard. When they smile, their eyes sparkle. We love to protect them and to tease them. We love to walk by the river, arm in arm, just to be with them. We love it most when they fall asleep in our arms. We cherish their very essence.

Is your wife your little ewe lamb?

You may feel uncomfortable with that imagery, and maybe it sounds chauvinistic to you. We're certainly not using it to describe relative levels of strength or ability. (*From Fred:* I know this from personal experience. My wife, Brenda, is an accomplished registered nurse and mother of four with firm views on everything. Yet in a tender moment when I told Brenda that I wanted to treat her like a "ewe lamb," she felt honored rather than offended.)

The Bible uses the term to capture a heavenly message. As Bathsheba was precious to Uriah, your wife is your precious one, your only one. She lives with you and lies in your arms. She's to be cherished, not because of what she does for you, but because of her essence, her value to God as a child born in His image. You've been entrusted with the priceless essence of another human soul, so precious to God that at the foundation of the world He planned to pay His dearest price to buy her back again.

Regardless of the current rubble in your marriage or the list of unmet conditions, you owe God to cherish that essence. When you look deeply enough into your wife's eyes, past the pain and hurts and fights, you can still find that little ewe lamb gazing back, hoping all things and trusting all things.

WHETHER YOU FEEL IT OR NOT

God entrusted your wife to you, and she placed herself in trust to you. How can we entrust such a valuable gift to some concept of cherishing based alone on wispy feelings? Christians like to say, "Love is not a feeling, it's a commitment." Well, this is the time to heed those words. We owe that love, despite our feelings.

In our society, we have "sensitivity training" and "cross-cultural enrichment" classes. We believe if we can only teach people the "right" feelings, they'll act correctly. In the Bible, however, God tells us the opposite: We're to first act correctly, and then right feelings will follow.

If you don't feel like cherishing, cherish anyway. Your right feelings will arrive soon enough..

Remember, the Bible says that God loved us while we were yet sinners. Clearly, loving the unlovely is a foundation of God's character, and *cherishing* the unlovely is its bedrock. Since Christ died for the church—the unlovely—and since our marriages should parallel Christ's relationship to the church, we have no excuse when we don't cherish our wives. God loved us before we were worthy; we can do nothing less for our wives.

carry the honor!

We've been talking about cherishing our wives, treating them with tenderness and holding them dear, despite our feelings. Let this final chapter be a reminder to experience the wonder at what she's given you and the enormous honor it is to carry her baton. Carry the honor nobly!

FROM FRED: HONOR HER FATHERS

As a father, I carry my daughter's baton. I remember when she was born. I remember cradling her when she was sick as a baby. Her fever was so high, her eyes rolled up into her head. After we rushed her to the doctor, she was so lethargic that she didn't feel the shot he gave her. I remember the time she broke her finger in the car door, and I held her close. I remember the time she won a part in a play, and I practiced with her again and again. I remember reviewing math flashcards with her night after night.

When the volleyball was spiked at her feet three times in a row at the family reunion, I held her close so she could hide her tears in my chest as she sobbed, "They all think I'm no good." I stayed close to her for the rest of the day, defending her honor and brazenly daring another spike against my "Peanut."

I labored over Laura's swimming strokes and sweated through my clothes when I taught her to ride her bike. I talked with her about junior high and how she was on the cusp of adolescence. I walked often to the altar with her, hand in hand, providing for her spiritual growth and understanding.

I learned to do her hair so she would always look nice, even when Mom was away. I bought her a few things she didn't really need—pictures, cashew nuts—just because I knew she would love them.

I carry the baton of care for my daughter, and no hip haircut, fast car, or sweet smile will trick it out of my hand. My investment is too great. My son-in-law will owe me big, and he'd better honor her!

When I asked for Brenda's baton from my father-in-law, he was on his deathbed. He strengthened from time to time, but we both knew his time on earth was nearly over. I entered his hospital room, much stronger than he, but far more frightened. I knew how he loved his daughter. I knew how he once held her and let her cry when she came home with a squirrel-cut instead of a haircut. I knew how he proudly gave her a used red Chevy Nova as a gift. I knew how he used to swim way out into the ocean and let her sit on him like a raft, floating merrily. I knew how he had diligently raised her in purity, keeping her in church and away from ribald influences on her life.

I asked for her hand, and then he said something to me that has remained engraved indelibly in my memory over the years: "Though I don't know you well, I know you're the kind of man that will do what you say. I know you'll take care of her." Never in my life had a man believed in me so, trusting my manhood and entrusting me with something so valuable. He gave his cherished only daughter to me, even while knowing he could never step back in to defend her if I didn't keep my word, that he would never be there to remind me of my promises, that he would never be there to put that sparkle back in her eye if I ever made it disappear.

I owe him because he trusted me. I owe him because he provided such a wonderful daughter to me. I owe him because of his great investment in her. When I see him again in heaven, I won't have to avert my eyes sheepishly in shame. He gave me the baton, and I *will* run well with it.

I also owe her other Father. He saved my life from sin and picked me up from the ash heap and set me among princes. He adopted me and gave me the strength for today and a bright hope for tomorrow. And he saved a precious ewe lamb for me, a pure one without spot or blemish, with sparkling eyes and a soft heart. He formed her in the womb and looked on with joy when she crawled and then walked and talked. He saw her sing "Throw Out the Lifeline" before Him as a member of the Singing Cousins. He sent His only Son to provide for her future, to protect her, and to bring her home to heaven safely. God isn't amused when I neglect to nurture a cherishing heart for her. He raised her and cherished her, and I must do the same.

REMEMBER WHAT SHE GIVES YOU

Your wife gave up her freedom for you. She relinquished her rights to seek happiness elsewhere. She exchanged this freedom for something she considered more valuable: your love and your word. Her dreams are tied up in you, dreams of sharing and communication and oneness.

She's pledged to be yours sexually. Her sexuality is her most guarded possession, her secret garden. She trusted you would be worthy of this gift, but you have cavalierly viewed sensual garbage, polluting and littering her garden. She deserves more, and you must honor that.

You must also cherish your wife because she shares her deepest secrets and longings with you. Brenda has told me stories she has told no one else. For instance, I know of a teasing word that, if I were to say it, would bring tears to her eyes instantly because of a trauma long ago. She's shared long-burning regrets and cried in my arms.

After years of marriage, I know what thrills her soul. I once entered a bookstore, leaving her waiting in the car. I purchased a book, passing over the "good customer" limit to earn a five-dollar gift certificate. The cashier asked whether she should apply it to my current purchase, but I said, "No, I'll save it for my wife. She'll be real excited about it."

Just then, Brenda walked in. I whispered to the clerk, "Watch this!" I turned and gave the gift certificate to Brenda. She squealed out loud and, giggling, said, "Ooh, this is great!" The cashier laughed with me.

You see, I know Brenda. She is my beloved, and I am hers. I know her deepest fears, her desires for the future, and what she absolutely can and can't handle. She risked much in opening up so wide, and I must have a cherishing heart for that.

When growing up, Brenda never feared anything because her dad was there. He never dishonored her, never shocked her, never frightened her, or let her down. She traded all that for a guy with a short fuse who yelled and argued and called her names. I'm the one who upset her stomach, forcing her into unpleasant in-law situations without trying to understand, at times making her cower in tears. She never traded for that. She traded for higher protection, but I gave her less.

Have you given less? Your wife risked much and traded much to marry you. Was it a good bargain for her?

HONOR HER HOPE

In my office I keep an eight-by-ten, black-and-white photo of Brenda when she was one year old. Her little eyes sparkle and are filled with the hope and joy of life, her mischievous smile apparent even then; her glowing, chubby cheeks radiating joy and a carefree spirit. That face is so full of expectations and wonder. I brought that infant picture to my office because it reminds me that I need to honor that hope.

I'm a man, and so I have a tendency to rebel. Life gets very hard sometimes, and work can drive me nearly out of my mind. I have four kids to provide for and a payroll to meet. I have church activities and sporting events and social obligations and on and on, and sometimes my heart begins to crumble. I hear my rebellious side scream for *my* rights and *my* way and *my* freedom, and sometimes I feel like jumping in the car and disappearing into the Great Northwest. Sad, but true.

But I can't when I think of Brenda. During long days of battle, her baby picture always reminds me that she's my little ewe lamb, always hopeful, always believing in me, always looking ahead for "us." I want the sparkling of those baby eyes shining in Brenda's eyes today, decades later. I *must* protect her beauty and grace and spotlessness.

You must honor your wife with a cherishing heart. God loved Uriah's love for Bathsheba. Does God love my love for Brenda? Does God love your love for your wife?

It doesn't matter what our wives look like, what they have or haven't done, or whether life has unfolded differently than we expected. We must honor and cherish them.

Clearly, life can unfold differently. *Very* differently. When Brenda and I first married, we were hoping to have four years together before having children, a time to build our relationship together. We'd known each other only seven months on our wedding day. In addition, Brenda's dad had died two months before the wedding. She moved three hours away from her hometown to start our life together. She was aching over her father, and she could not support her mother in her grief from that distance. We were searching for a church and had no friends. She had a new job, and I was fairly new in mine. In commission sales, money was tight. After expenses, my first year's income was below the poverty line, and I also had fifteen thousand dollars' worth of school and business debt. We were also reeling under in-law problems.

As I've said, our marriage nearly crumbled under that pressure. Then, of all things, Brenda announced she was pregnant shortly after our first wedding anniversary.

After Jasen was born, the boy wouldn't sleep at night. We tried every trick, including letting him cry for long periods, sometimes for hours. Our discouragement was nearly debilitating. Confused, Brenda couldn't take another blow. Life hadn't turned out as we'd hoped, and too often I didn't have a cherishing heart.

Gratefully, I'd just made my "eat gravel" stand with God in front of the refrigerator. Reading about Uriah for the first time, I began to see Brenda in a new way. I began to cherish her, despite the circumstances. I began to treat her with tenderness, holding her dear in spite of my feelings. I decided to get up with my son every time he awoke at night even though Brenda didn't work outside the home after Jasen was born. Logically, since she didn't work and could rest at different times during the day, she should have been the one to get up. By some standards, I should have said, "C'mon, you're a big girl now. Pull yourself up by your bootstraps and get tough!" But *anyone* could say that. She could have gotten that kind of treatment as a single woman.

But she was married to me, and she was my little ewe lamb. I cherished her, helping her out when she needed it most. How could I do that? She was no longer the person I thought I married, and I didn't always feel tender toward her, but I did it because it was right. The tender feelings followed later.

A Promise

During that same period, I noticed a peculiar thing. The physical drain of nursing, the unsettled sleep at night (she would get up and nurse, then hand Jasen to me), and the psychological exhaustion wasted Brenda. If she awoke in the morning and stumbled down to a dirty kitchen, she was immediately discouraged and had difficulty starting her day. Her courage melted; she found it easier just to stay in her pajamas all day. Life seemed dark and dreary.

I didn't like my ewe lamb to start her day like this. Yes, I could have asked Brenda to shape up, grit her teeth, and push harder. I could have reminded her that she wasn't living up to my expectations. Instead, I made a promise to my wife that I would never go to bed with the kitchen dirty.

I knew what that promise would cost me. Because of her exhaustion, it meant she would often head off to bed and leave me alone to do all the dishes and scrub all the pans. It meant that often she would be asleep when I got to bed, and I would miss out on sex. It meant that I would miss out on precious sleep, but I also knew that I could cherish my ewe lamb in ways she never thought possible. I never broke my promise.

I cherished Brenda when the feelings weren't there, and my feelings returned. Eventually, she grew to the woman she is today. She's *everything* I knew she would be. But guess what? She's also more. She saw my cherishing heart and stopped talking divorce. These days, when I speak about God's Word and about living by His standards, I have credibility with her because I've proven myself with her in the unloveliest of times.

YOUR SONG

Our final word for you: If cherishing is anything, it's loving your wife for who she is *this day,* not some other day down the line. It's making allowances for all the surprises and inconsistencies that were hidden until life spun her in its new direction.

Your wife has a heart that still beats like a little lamb's heart, a heart that still skips through meadows of hope and desire, longing for love. It may be difficult to see. Maybe her father was an alcoholic or an abuser who didn't protect her. Maybe she isn't much of a Christian. Maybe she was promiscuous before meeting you.

Maybe so. But we know some other things are also true.

In trust to you, she *did* forsake her individual freedom, believing you would provide love and protection.

She's God's little ewe lamb regardless of the pain and sin she's been through, and *He* has entrusted her to you.

Can you see into her soul? Does your heart warm to the task? Is there anything more noble than making a solemn promise to cherish your one and only?

Be content with the wife of your youth. If she isn't all you'd hoped for, remember that God graced you with this ewe lamb. Can you make a commitment to cherish her today? If so, let your mind be transformed by the Word. Let your song be Solomon's Song:

> *How beautiful you are, my darling.*
> > *Oh, how beautiful!*
> > *Your eyes behind your veil are doves…*
> *Your lips are like a scarlet ribbon,*
> > *your mouth is lovely…*
> *All beautiful you are, my darling;*
> > *there is no flaw in you…*
> *You have stolen my heart, my sister, my bride;*
> > *you have stolen my heart*
> > *with one glance of your eyes…*
> *How delightful is your love, my sister, my bride!…*
> *Your head crowns you like Mount Carmel.*
> > *Your hair is like royal tapestry;*
> > *the king is held captive by its tresses.*
> *How beautiful you are and how pleasing,*
> > *O love, with your delights.*
> > > *(Song of Songs 4:1,3,7,9-10; 7:5-6)*

The Heart of a Woman

Cherishing appears in many ways. One of the simplest we heard was from Frances, who said, "I'm always thrilled to see my hubby, even when he's far across the church."

Deena said, "I'm trying very hard to speak only good things of him and to build him up. I'm trying not to cut him down even when joking, being sure to consider his feelings as much as my own these days."

Brenda said, "Cherishing often manifests itself in simple, daily things more than big romantic things. Things like doing my jobs at home and cutting finances when necessary. It should also show in my obvious desire to be with Fred all the time."

These daily acts create feelings of cherishing and tenderness, but comparison can tear out a man's heart. Guys compare the neighborhoods they live in, the cars they drive, the people they socialize with, and the families they come from. Many men struggle with this to some degree, but most will never reveal this side of themselves to their wives, even when asked. They feel trapped by their fate.

It isn't what part of town we live in that decides our fate in the end. Generally, that's something we can't control. What we *can* control is how much hope we give to our spouse. What a husband needs is someone to look deeply into his eyes to remind him that his wife loves him and God loves him.

When Ellen told her husband that she is content to live on the income he has provided without complaint or comparison, he was fulfilled. To Ellen, that essence is priceless. "My goal in life, next to loving and obeying God, has been to love and learn about my husband and to help him be fulfilled and to enjoy living life together."

If Brenda compared Fred to some of her high-school peers, she would find that he's doing quite well. If she financially compared him to the folks at church, she would probably find her family somewhere in the middle. If she compared him to his Stanford peers, he'd probably rank as a scraggly, under-achieving dog. But that's how comparison works. It's relative and, therefore, unreliable.

Who cares anyway? "The essential thing I owe Fred is faithfulness and trustworthiness," she said. "No one else in his life has proven completely true in these areas. I'm absolutely committed that although we may differ some-times, I'll always be faithful to him. I will stay his one and only."

Brenda respects what she's found and treats the weak spots tenderly. When she's cherishing him like this, it becomes easy for Fred to cherish her in return.

Today you may not feel cherished because of your husband's sexual sin. When we asked women if they could cherish their husbands if they found them stuck in sexual sin, their answers were shaky.

Ellen said, "I would try. I would have such great sorrow and disappointment. It would take some time and much prayer to cherish him fully. I would ask God to help me to cherish him as I should. It would be very difficult. Not difficult to love him, but difficult to cherish him, especially if he had a problem and hadn't shared it early on. The trust would be broken, and I would feel that he didn't trust me or he would have shared the problem so we could get help."

Frances used the key word "respect." "It would be very difficult to respect and trust him." Her cherishing heart would be on life support, since respect is the essence of cherishing.

Cathy said, "After the initial shock, and if he showed a true desire to purify himself, and after healing from the Lord, I think I would still cherish him. After all, we all have weaknesses and sin encroaching into our lives."

Andrea said, "Because we've already dealt with this once, I can truly appre-ciate the incredible hold that the sexual-impurities problem has. The Bible is very clear that all sin is sin; one sin isn't better than another. The past year or two, God has really been working on me not to judge people and their sins, but rather to sympathize with them and pray with them. So I would hope I would look at it the same way with my husband and still cherish him for who he is."

In the end, women still must cherish their husbands. No sin frees husbands or wives from that responsibility.

We all struggle with sin. We all struggle with sacrificing our own visible kingdoms for God's invisible kingdom. To whatever extent your husband has won his battle against sexual sin, he deserves extra respect. But even in defeat he needs your respect. Cherish him.

Find your husband's deepest essence and cherish him sacrificially as God did on the cross. Respect and honor him, however unrespectable he may seem. Fully give yourself to him. Look into his soul and sing:

> My lover [my husband] is radiant and ruddy,
>   outstanding among ten thousand.
> His head is purest gold;
>   his hair is wavy
>   and black as a raven....
> His mouth is sweetness itself;
>   he is altogether lovely.
> This is my lover, this is my friend....
> I belong to my lover,
>   and his desire is for me....
> Let us go early to the vineyards...
>   there I will give you my love.
> The mandrakes send out their fragrance,
>   and at our door is every delicacy,
> both new and old,
>   that I have stored up for you, my lover.
>   (Song of Songs 5:10-11,16; 7:10,12-13)

the final step

At one time, maybe these lovely words from Song of Solomon described your marriage, but today they seem as foreign as Greek or Latin.

As for the purposes of God in your marriage, perhaps you haven't even considered them in a while. Maybe you're experiencing a semblance of peace at home? After all, if the garage is fairly well organized, the bills are getting paid, and you're able to play a round of golf from time to time, why question things too much?

Well, you should, because a great marriage is more than those kinds of things. Are you bored with your marriage? Do you have a truce in your marital relationship but no deep oneness? Does male leadership in marriage confuse you and frustrate your wife? Is your wife failing to fulfill you sexually?

Great marriages may seem rare these days, but God didn't intend it that way. By God's way of thinking, a vibrant, cherishing relationship is quite normal and should be quite common because, believe it or not, you already have what it takes to walk faithfully like Uriah:

> His divine power has given us everything we need for life
> and godliness through our knowledge of him who called us
> by his own glory and goodness. Through these he has given
> us his very great and precious promises, so that through
> them you may participate in the divine nature and escape

the corruption in the world caused by evil desires. (2 Peter 1:3-4)

You and your wife already have what it takes to sculpt a glorious image of Christ's relationship to the church, a masterpiece so lovely it will draw men and women to Christ simply by their looking at the two of you together.

Five hundred years ago, when Michelangelo was lauded for his famous sculptural masterpiece *David*, he refused the praise, replying that he had really done nothing at all. He said that the image of David was in that rock from the time of creation—that his hands were merely the tools to chip away the excess stone that revealed the beauty placed there by God eons ago.

Like Michelangelo, you must chip away the stony "flesh" and attitudes that overlay your marriage and block the beauty God placed there when you were married.

Sadly, too often much of the excess stone overlays the husband's part of the sculpture, leaving the wife to struggle with less than she'd been promised in both the marriage bed and her home. Perhaps the husband's false intimacy found in pornography and masturbation has pushed out the true intimacy that should have been in the marriage from the beginning.

Has your guilt stunted the development of a prayer life together? Has your guilt kept you from seeking God's face and searching through the convicting Word of God? Perhaps such guilt has left you grumpy, and your relationship with God has wilted like dry prairie grass under a broiling late-August sun. If so, your marriage probably hasn't fared much better. Like many guys, your marital problems may not stop at your sexual sin. Take a look at the following letter:

My husband has bought into the lie that "all men look" because they are visual. He says it is impossible for any real man not to look at the babe in the string bikini. He threatened me with divorce if I don't stop nagging him, and he says if I'm looking for a man who doesn't notice other women, I'm going to be terribly hurt for a long time.

Listen carefully to her pain as she continues:

I am sick to my stomach to think that, for the rest of my life, I will be robbed from having fullness from my marriage. Because this bothers me so much and my husband is so sick of being reminded, he does it even more! Can you imagine? Everywhere I go with my husband I know I can't keep his attention—*nowhere!*

Do you notice that this guy is committing two different sins? While the sexual sin is obvious, he's also guilty of arrogant leadership and rude responses to his wife's thoughts and feelings. Even if this husband reverses course and purifies his eyes, his leadership style will continue to trample her heart in other areas of their relationship.

If sexual sin is not your only issue, you may be hurting your wife in a myriad of ways, from ignoring her pleas to telling her to shut up—and this can hurt your battle for sexual purity. These sins have consequences, too. For instance, you may get your sexual sin under control and find your sexual desire for your wife increasing, only then to find that her desire for *you* is DOA because of the many times you've trampled her heart over the years.

Or your wife may respond like this one did when her husband joined a couple of guys to study *Every Man's Battle Workbook:* "Oh, so you've formed a little club to go through your 'sex books' together? I hope you have fun with all your perverted little friends!"

Disrespect and resentment permeate this wife's feelings for her husband. Where did they come from? Perhaps his insensitive leadership crushed her love for him.

We know that relationships can be complicated, and everything is not cut and dried. It doesn't help that we men are ill-equipped to understand women and relationships—even when we *think* we understand and we *think* we are doing well.

Having said that, I want you to know that you are a warrior of the Lord God Almighty. The battle for purity lies before you, and victory is yours for the taking. God is with you, and make no mistake, together you stand as a formidable duo on the battlefield.

You can—and will—win this battle. But what happens next? You'll need a comrade standing at your shoulder as you build true intimacy into your marriage. That person must be your wife, your helpmate.

You love her. We know you want to cherish your wife and want her to *feel* cherished. You want her to become everything you ever dreamed she could be.

We also know that, deep down, you're suspecting that if you could just lead right and cherish her well, she would truly blossom in your home and help cement your victory over sexual sin for the rest of your life.

I know that the more Brenda blossoms, the more my heart longs to do well as a Christian. And the more I do well as a Christian, the more she blossoms.

So as you finish *Every Man's Battle* and begin building the defense perimeters into your life, Steve and I urge you to take one more step. Pick up and read a copy of *Every Man's Marriage* (formerly titled *Every Woman's Desire*), our detailed guide that teaches you how to cherish your wife. This is a book that answers the question: What is every woman's desire? Answer: A husband who will honor and cherish her. You'll learn how to do that in *Every Man's Marriage*. From the beginning, we've always intended *Every*

Man's Marriage to be read along with *Every Man's Battle*. In fact, in many ways, Steve and I feel that *Every Man's Marriage* is the most important book in the Every Man series. We've heard from readers that they feel it is our best book. We share these comments only to underscore the passion we have for building strong marriages.

In light of that passion, we'll close by returning one last time to some thoughts from an earlier passage. It's time to rise up, friend. Be one of the King's mighty men. Uriah's faithfulness was complete. Isn't it time for yours to be complete too?

After all, you are saved, and you've sworn your life to the purposes of God. You've sworn your life to someone else too. You promised before family and friends to honor and cherish your wife, abandoning all others. You gave your word that she would have more from marriage than she would have as a single woman. Are you consumed by this commitment? Consumed enough to live faithfully and to cherish her completely? Consumed enough to read one more book to make sure you know exactly what God wants of you?

Pick up a copy of *Every Man's Marriage*. Read it once, and then read it again with your wife. She may point out some things you've missed or haven't seen, but that's okay. She wants the best for you—and your marriage.

After all, *that* is every woman's desire.

the rest of the story

FROM FRED

Ten years. I can scarcely believe it's been that long since *Every Man's Battle* first hit the presses, but it's true, which brings up an interesting question: what's a decade worth?

It all depends on what you do with it. Near the end of my third decade of life, the rubble was piling up at my feet. I couldn't look God in the eye anymore, and I was betraying Brenda with my gaze and my mind. Furthermore, I was compromising the spiritual protection over my home, living in terror that one day I'd pass this suffocating pattern of sin onto my kids.

My firstborn, Jasen, was already on the scene, a cute little squirt, one great big ball of herky-jerky, drooling action. At times he'd amble awkwardly over to me with a drippy pacifier somehow loosely held in his mouth, while shooting me a goofy grin as big as the moon. Though he couldn't speak, I knew exactly what his eyes were saying: *Daddy, you are my hero. I want to grow up to be just like you!*

Many times I'd simply sweep him into my arms and tickle him because I loved him so. But on other occasions when we were home alone together, I'd burst into hopeless tears. *No!* I'd beg inside. *Please don't become like me, Son! I'm not your hero. If I were, I would save you from this prison, but I can't even save myself. How will I ever save you?*

That's where I stood at the end of that decade, hopeless and aimless amid the dusty debris of my inner life. I'm grateful that God waded into this mess, challenging me to change the direction of my family tree and chasing me incessantly with Luke 6:46: "Why do you call me, 'Lord, Lord,' and do not do what I say?"

As this devastating question began to seize my heart, I grappled hard over the costs and the possibilities of fighting back. Winning sounded great, but the battle seemed too difficult and confusing. I waffled over this issue for months until my exasperated Father in heaven spoke this chilling challenge into my heart: *Are you going to drive the stake into the ground right here and change the destiny of your family tree, or will you be leaving the job for someone who's better than you, somewhere down the line?*

My heart writhed in grinding torment. Would I face up to the raging war at hand? The choice was as simple as it was stark: I could either man up and pick a fight with this brutal sexual taskmaster, or I could drift into the rabble of adulterous Stoeker men and spend the rest of my days merely posing as a man, as they had.

The time for posing was over. My family's destiny depended upon it, as did my manhood. Just a few days after God's challenge, I engaged the battle for keeps while driving down Merle Hay Road, slamming my fists into the steering wheel and driving that stake firmly into the ground.

A new decade dawned for me that day. What would that decade be worth? Everything.

During those years, I began providing to my wife what God calls every man to deliver in marriage. Brenda put it this way:

> I feel incredible security knowing that I'm married to a man
> who keeps his eyes to himself. Even after four babies and
> twenty-four years of aging together, I live unthreatened by

any women around me. Fred loves me for me and is very satisfied with who I am and what I've become.

When my husband prays, I'm confident that nothing is hindering his connection with God. If I knew of dark, hidden areas, I'd have no faith that his prayers would even rise to the ceiling, but I've seen how a pure man's prayer packs a spiritual punch.

My confidence in Fred's spiritual protection is unbounded. I never wonder if there are open cracks in our spiritual defenses where the Enemy can slip into our lives. Christianity is not a game to Fred, and image means nothing. He'd rather *be* a Christian than seem like one.

Fred has every right to make the decisions for our family because it's God's plan, but even if it weren't, he's earned that right through his actions. He's proven in battle that his commitment to the Lord and his love for his family are the highest priorities in his life, and we simply rest in his strength.

This normal, godly pattern leaves everyone flourishing, and this wouldn't be possible if blatant sin were clogging things up. I know who Fred is, and in the secret places of life, I know where he will not go. (Brenda Stoeker, *Every Heart Restored,* page 189)

That's not all. I saw early signs that my kids were free from the generational patterns of sexual sin. When Jasen neared puberty, he turned away from some pornography brought to school by his classmates. For the first time in generations, a Stoeker walked away from porn!

By the end of the decade, my relationship with God was soaring. We'd gotten so close that He entrusted me with leading the intercession team at church, and just as that decade came to a close, the Lord began nudging me to write *Every Man's Battle.* Unbelievable.

Now another ten years have come and gone, and we're celebrating the tenth anniversary of a book that's traveling around the world, declaring its message of freedom in more than twenty languages. A second great decade in a row, no doubt about it.

But let's face it, my friend. When it comes to the rest of the story in any man's life, it's not about the books written or the dollars of product sold or the promotions earned or any other milestones passed along the way. What counts is how you and your character have changed. The impact of those changes will cascade down through your family tree, and then ripple out through the body of Christ as a testimony of grace, impacting *God's* family too.

So what's a decade worth? It's worth exactly the testimony you write with it, which may be priceless. Testimonies are powerful things, as Scripture reminds us: "Worship God! For the testimony of Jesus is the spirit of prophecy" (Revelation 19:10).

A testimony reveals what's possible in our lives as men. The original language for the word *testimony* can be translated "to do again," and that's where its power lies. The moment you read or hear a testimony, the Holy Spirit shifts the spiritual atmosphere. Faith explodes in your heart, and hope swirls throughout your soul: *If God can do this in that guy's life, then God can do it in mine.* The power of testimony lies in that stirring of faith, and the Holy Spirit needs only a little faith to duplicate the testimony in you and work victory throughout your life.

I've heard from thousands of guys how our testimonies charged their faith and changed their lives. But some still doubt victory is possible, and now and then I'll receive an email like this: "Fred, you've lived another decade on the front lines of the battle. In your book you seemed so certain that victory could last. Are you still winning the battle?"

I can faithfully report that I am *still* winning and victory *has* been complete. In fact, during the last twenty years, I haven't once searched the magazines or newspapers or surfed the cable channels or the Web for sensual sights to lust over, from lingerie ads to exercise shows to sensuous movies. It's not that I *can't* stumble anymore. I simply don't. If you really get after it in this battle, your mind *will* be transformed. Don't be deceived. The temptations actually *do* fade, and the battle *will* change forever.

Sure, some guys claim victory isn't possible. Megan told me, "My husband bristles at the concept of being able to eradicate sexual impurity in a man's life. Reduce it, perhaps, but eliminate it? Never."

But it *is* possible. I know, because I live there, and what's more, God can do it again in your life and in the lives of your sons, just like He did in my family.

A SON WHO MAKES ME PROUD

Perhaps you'd like to know what happened to Jasen over these past ten years too. You already know he started well, turning away from porn that first time. But did he keep turning away over the years?

I'll cut right to the chase, comparing his first year out of college to mine. When I was twenty-three, I was sleeping regularly with three different girls and essentially engaged to marry two of them. When Jasen was twenty-three, I watched him take his newly minted wife in to his arms at his wedding and kiss a girl for the very first time, ever.

What's more, he never got hooked on porn and masturbation along the way, and he never left a girl worse off for having known him while dating. (He shares how he managed this in his book *Hero,* which I co-wrote with him.) His life and marriage are a testament to God's faithfulness for every man out there who still wonders whether sexual purity is really possible in today's culture. God did all that for us in a single generation, and He can do it again for you.

Now, that doesn't mean you won't have a fight on your hands, even if you *do* get your eyes under control by the end of six weeks, like I did. Sure, those were wonderful days, an awesome time of many glorious victories, and my relationship with God blossomed in wonderful ways in the weeks and months that followed. Compared to the first six weeks of heavy head-on war, the rest of the battle seemed like mop-up duty.

But I still had to deal with stiff pockets of resistance. Though my eyes were finally under control, for a time my mind was still conjuring up sexual fantasies, and while my masturbation habit had been weakened severely by my covenant with my eyes, it would still be another three years before I masturbated for the last time—even though I was married and getting all the sex I wanted.

Surprised? Don't be. Masturbation, while obviously sexual in nature, is more than a sexual issue. Sure, there are sexual triggers to masturbation, like watching a double feature of *American Pie* and *American Pie 2.* But there are also emotional triggers, like the stress of work or old emotional wounds from our fathers.

In my estimation, the emotional triggers to masturbate are often stronger than the sexual triggers, meaning that your masturbation habit may actually be more of an emotional addiction than a sexual one. That's why guys can cut the eye candy and still find themselves addicted to masturbation.

The important point is that my defeats during this time were critical to my eventual victory. Every loss taught me more about myself, my emotional triggers, and where my defenses were down. I learned to embrace the losses, seek God, fight on, and win.

My book *Tactics* will help you with this part of the battle. It may be part of our Every Man's youth trilogy, but *Tactics* was actually written to help any man work through the latter stages of this battle when facing various pockets of resistance. Let me share what Randy, age fifty-two, found in *Tactics*:

> I think *Tactics* is even more powerful than *Every Man's Battle,* which is saying something. I learned so much about my physical and mental makeup, but the one thing I cherished most was learning how you worship the Lord in song before praying. I've had very rewarding conversations with our Lord lately as a result. Through this one book, you've taught me more about having devotional times with God than anybody else I know.

And that's the whole point of sexual purity. It's not only about guarding your eyes and starving your mind. It's about deepening your connection with God and being forged as a man. This battle was designed to prove to yourself and to the world that you're man enough to be everything your Christian label promises you'll be. Jon is now that kind of man:

> I was seven when my brother and I began modeling with a Christian agency whose goal was to place missionaries in the advertising world. After high school, I won an elite contest, signed with a New York City agency, and began to travel extensively. At nineteen I was continually surrounded by nudity on the set and in our coed changing rooms. The sensual photo shoots kept my mind racing, and one-night stands became the norm for me. My view of sex and relationships was quickly warped.
>
> Before long I became a promoter in the club scene in Manhattan, creating buzz and filling clubs with hip pretty

people. I did it well, setting them up with whatever they wanted but basically pimping them for my gain. As a kid I'd been trained to know God, but I couldn't see what I'd become. I was certainly no missionary.

Through something of a miracle, on a trip home I found *Every Man's Battle* lying on my nightstand. I was frozen by the words and instantly knew they were all true. While I wasn't following the Lord at the time, I felt compelled to apply the principles. That began a cascade of change in my heart that continues to this day.

Soon I was bouncing my eyes from billboards, turning the other way while changing clothes with girls, getting photographers to change racy shoots, and avoiding magazine racks, even walking past them backward. I didn't care anymore how I looked—I was committed to keeping my eyes pure.

After talking with two guys at a YWAM conference, God convinced me I needed to quit modeling. It felt crazy, but I knew it was my only way to complete freedom. It was also time to learn to do relationships the right way. I cut off communication with the women in my past, and I haven't touched or kissed a woman in a sensual way since.

God also showed me I needed a community of believers. I joined a Christian study program called Transit and was soon asked to go to Southeast Asia with a small team to rescue women from human trafficking. I prayed about it and asked a friend for advice. "Did God tell you don't go?" he asked. "No." "Is your heart broken over what's happening there?" "Yes." "Then that's your answer."

So I went. In Cambodia my transformed heart, its

natural heroism springing to life and now emboldened by the trust God gave me with this special mission, burned to help the prostitutes and sex slaves. In Bangkok we went to an open-air market called the night bazaar, a two-lane street lined by strip clubs three to five stories high, with bars at street level and sex rooms above. Women and girls pole danced inside. The streets were filled with middle-aged Western men with twentysomething Thai women on their arms and teenagers walking slowly back and forth, peeking into the clubs. I felt overwhelming rage and nearly vomited from disgust. Tourists of all ages and nationalities strolled the streets while promoters tried to lure them into the bars. I wanted to punch them, until the Lord reminded me of New York. Except for God, I was no different from these guys.

I've never sensed such wretched oppression anywhere, and prayer had never seemed so crucial to me. My friend and I teamed up each night to prayer-walk the red-light district while the women on our team went into the clubs to talk with the girls. We prayed out loud the whole way, looking like a couple tourists talking together. During the days, we heard from teams and met the women rescued the night before. It was beyond amazing. Rather than using God's daughters, I was now defending them, and I'd finally become that missionary God dreamed I'd be.

The battle for purity is also about becoming your wife's hero and not her nightmare, and proving you're man enough to make your commitments to her stick. That's why you must ask your wife soon to join you on this great battlefield. She's the woman you're fighting for, and you need her support.

But that support won't be automatic. Humble yourself. Toss out the pretense and quit posing as someone you aren't, insisting she keep this news away from her friends at church. She needs a support group, and she'll need to talk with others like her. Quit shifting the blame, sneering that her weight gain has caused your horrific sin. Get real, man. You were addicted long before you even met her, and if she's not as attractive as she used to be, it's likely because you haven't disciplined your eyes to love only her.

Stop dictating the terms, like, *I'll do anything except go to counseling.* Stop making demands, like, *Just shut up with the questions and stick to praying.* You've crushed her soul, my friend. She has a right to ask questions, and she needs counsel to heal. Be a man. You made the mess, so clean it up, whatever it takes. Go to the counselor. Answer her questions.

Drop the self-serving lies, like, *Men are visual, and you'll just have to get used to it.* No, she doesn't need to get used to it. You need to get used to living Christianly, like being captivated by her love and being satisfied by her breasts alone (see Proverbs 5:18-19).

She is not your enemy. In fact, she'll be your greatest ally—if only you'll let her in. Open the door and start reading *Every Heart Restored* together, because if you expect to stand as one in this battle, she'll need to understand male sexuality far better than she does, and you'll need to understand just how cruelly you've hurt her. Give her a copy of *The Healing Choice,* a book Brenda wrote with Susan Allen, which will help her get closer to God than she's ever been. *The Healing Choice* will also help her find women to support her on this rocky rugged journey, through a wonderful ministry called Avenue.

COMING CLEAN

I understand your fears. I've stood alone with my secrets amid the dusty rubble, and I know it's scary to reveal them. What will happen when you do? I don't know for certain, but I *do* know that hope always dawns in the midst of the storm, just as it did for Ray:

I'm at a crossroads to come clean with my wife, but I'm afraid to be honest with her because I fear full disclosure will be the death sentence to our marriage. Still, I sense real hope right now because today is the first day I have cried in repentance before God, and today I know this sin has kept me from being the man Jesus wants me to be.

Today could also be the first day of a new decade of life for you and your family. What will that decade be worth? Perhaps everything, just as it was for me, and just as it's shaping up for Bill and Amber. Here's what Amber had to say:

Several months ago I was browsing through some of my older books and ran across *Every Heart Restored*. I perused some of the pages and realized just how much I had healed. When I first read your book, there were many parts that seemed like salt on an open wound, but they don't exact the same emotional toll now. I was overwhelmed with gratitude toward God. I began weeping in prayer with an inconsolable burden for others who were going through that same trauma I barely lived through back then.

I want to thank you for your openness and candor on this issue, as you've allowed me to see past my hurt and reopen my spiritual ears to God. Not only have I been totally restored from the hurts of the past, but our marriage is now better than it's ever been.

I attend a large popular church, but this ugly phenomenon of pornography can lie beneath any church's veneer, trapping those who are ashamed to admit to it. I told our pastor that our church should start support groups for those stuck on these sinking boats, and he agreed. Oddly enough, he wants Bill and me to lead them. Well, maybe that's not so odd.

I have gone from death to life—from choking down handfuls of sleeping pills day after day, because it hurt too much emotionally to stay awake, to living with an exuberant overwhelming desire to help others receive the same healing God gave me. Even if you had been able to reach only one hurting family, I promise you that all your efforts would've been worth it. My family is so indebted to yours.

Every testimony begins on a single day, much like this day, my friend. Make some choices. Let God wade in. Step out of your rubble, and step into His light. Engage the battle at His side. After all, it's a brand new decade. Take up your life, and write Him a testimony.

This time around, make it one for the ages.

workbook

questions you may have about this workbook

What will the *Every Man's Battle Workbook* do for me?

This workbook will guide you through some serious Bible study, an intense examination of your personal life, and an honest application of biblical truth to help you win the war on sexual temptation and live a pure life God's way.

You'll find realistic help straight from God's Word for actively training your eyes and your mind to increasingly see and think according to God's standards.

Is this workbook enough or do I also need to read *Every Man's Battle*?

Included in the studies you'll find a few featured excerpts from *Every Man's Battle,* each one marked at the beginning and end by this symbol: 🔔. But you really do need to read along in *Every Man's Battle* to truly get the most out of this companion workbook. (You'll find the appropriate chapters to read listed at the beginning of each weekly study.)

The lessons look long. Do I need to work through everything in each one?

This workbook is designed to promote your thorough exploration of all the content, but you may find it best to focus your time and discussion on some sections and questions more than others.

To help your pacing, we've designed the workbook so it can most easily be used in either an eight-week or twelve-week approach.

- *For the eight-week track,* simply follow along with the basic organization already set up with the eight different weekly lessons.
- *For the twelve-week track,* the lessons labeled Weeks Two, Five, Six, and Seven can be divided into two parts (you'll see the dividing place marked in the text).

(In addition, of course, you may decide to follow at a different pace—faster or slower—whether you're going through the workbook individually or as part of a group.)

Above all, keep in mind that the purpose of this workbook is to help guide you in specific life-application of the biblical truths taught in *Every Man's Battle.* The wide questions included in each weekly study are meant to help you approach this practical application from different angles and with personal reflection and self-examination. Allowing adequate time to prayerfully reflect on each question will be much more valuable for you than rushing through the workbook.

How do I bring together a small group to go through this workbook?
You'll get far more out of this workbook if you're able to go through it together with a small group of like-minded men. And what do you do if you don't know of any group that's going through this workbook? Start such a group of your own!

If you take a copy of the book *Every Man's Battle,* plus a copy of this companion workbook, and show them to the Christian men you know, you'll be surprised at how many will indicate interest in joining you for exploring this topic together. And it doesn't require a long commitment from them. The workbook is clearly set up so you complete one lesson per week and finish in only eight weeks—or, if you'd like to proceed at a little slower pace, you can follow the instructions provided for covering the exact same content in a twelve-week track.

Your once-per-week meeting could happen during the lunch hour one day at work, in the early morning before work begins, on a weekday evening, or even a Saturday morning. The location could be an office or meeting room at work, a room at a club or restaurant, a classroom at church, or someone's basement or den at home. Choose a location where your discussion won't be overhead by others, so the men are comfortable in sharing candidly and freely.

This workbook follows a simple design that's easy to use. First, each man in the group completes a week's lesson on his own. Then, when you come together that week, you discuss together the group questions provided under the Every Man's TALK heading in each week's lesson. Of course, if you have time, you can also discuss at length any of the other questions or topics in that week's lesson; we guarantee the men in your group will find these to be worth exploring. And they're likely as well to have plenty of their own related questions to bring up for discussion.

It's best if one person in your group is designated as the group's facilitator. This person is *not* a lecturer or teacher, but simply has the responsibility to keep the discussion moving and to ensure that each man in the group has an opportunity to fully join in.

At the beginning, remind the men of the simple ground rule that anything shared in the group *stays* in the group—everything's confidential. This will help the men feel safer about sharing honestly and openly in an environment of trust.

Finally we encourage you during each meeting together to allow time for prayer—conversational, short-sentence prayers expressed in honesty before God. Many men don't feel comfortable praying aloud before others, so in an understanding way, do all you can to help them overcome that barrier.

where are we?

Before men experience victory over sexual sin, they're hurting and confused. Why can't I win at this? they think. As the fight wears on and the losses pile higher, we begin to doubt everything about ourselves, even our salvation. At best, we think that we're deeply flawed. At worst, evil persons. We feel very alone, since men speak little of these things.

But we're not alone. Many men have fallen into their own sexual pits.

—from chapter 3 in *Every Man's Battle*

📖 EVERY MAN'S TRUTH

(Your Personal Journey into God's Word)

As you begin this study, ask for the Holy Spirit's help in hearing and obeying His personal words for you. Read and meditate upon the following Bible passages, which have to do with God's holiness and His call to purity. Let the Lord remind you that He is calling you to purity because He has your best interest at heart. Also remember that He delights in you—as one who is made in His image and growing into His likeness, day by day.

You have heard that it was said, "Do not commit adultery."
But I tell you that anyone who looks at a woman lustfully
has already committed adultery with her in his heart.
(Matthew 5:27-28)

Who will bring any charge against those whom God has
chosen? It is God who justifies. Who is he that condemns?
Christ Jesus, who died—more than that, who was raised
to life—is at the right hand of God and is also interceding for us. Who shall separate us from the love of Christ?
Shall trouble or hardship or persecution or famine or
nakedness or danger or sword?… No, in all these things
we are more than conquerors through him who loved us.
For I am convinced that neither death nor life, neither
angels nor demons, neither the present nor the future,
nor any powers, neither height nor depth, nor anything
else in all creation, will be able to separate us from the
love of God that is in Christ Jesus our Lord. (Romans
8:33-35,37-39)

"Come now, let us reason together,"
    says the LORD.
"Though your sins are like scarlet,
    they shall be as white as snow;
though they are red as crimson,
    they shall be like wool." (Isaiah 1:18)

1. What do Jesus' words tell you about His deep concern for your
   thought life?

2. What comfort do you take in Paul's words to the Roman believers? How does this passage relate to your feelings of guilt when you've given in to lust?

3. When it comes to a believer's sin, how would you distinguish between rebellion and immaturity? What is God's attitude toward us as we grow—and as we stumble—in our attempts to walk in holiness with Him? (Think about your relationship to your own children, if you have them.)

4. "White as snow" is the prophet's imagery for God's holiness. To what extent do you long for holiness and purity in your life? How are Isaiah's words hopeful to you?

☑ EVERY MAN'S CHOICE
(Questions for Personal Reflection and Examination)

📖 Pursuing sexual integrity is a controversial topic. We've been ridiculed by the world's sophisticates who find God's standard ridiculous and confining. That's fine with us, because we have a bigger concern—you. You're in a tough position. You live in a world awash with sensual images available twenty-four hours a day in a variety of mediums: print, television, videos, the Internet—even phones. 📖

📖 After teaching on the topic of male sexual purity in Sunday school, I was approached one day by a man who said, "I always thought that since I was a man I would not be able to control my roving eyes. I didn't know it could be any other way." 📖

5. Why do you think pursuing sexual integrity is such a controversial topic? How realistic is this pursuit for you?

6. How aware are you of the sensual images all around you? What has been your way of dealing with—or *not* dealing with—this bombardment of sexuality on a daily basis?

7. Have you ever considered your roving eye to be uncontrollable? In the past, when have you been most likely to lose control? What has helped you to exercise control?

📖 EVERY MAN'S WALK
(Your Guide to Personal Application)

> 📖 Steve: I can't tell you what her face looked like; nothing above the neckline registered with me that morning. My eyes feasted on this banquet of glistening flesh as she passed on my left, and they continued to follow her lithe figure as she continued jogging southbound. I turned my head further and further, craning my neck to capture every possible moment for my mental video camera.
>
> Then *blam!* I might still be marveling at this remarkable specimen of female athleticism if my Mercedes hadn't plowed into a Chevelle that had come to a complete stop in my lane. 📖

> 📖 Fred: There was a monster lurking about, and it surfaced each Sunday morning when I settled in my comfy La-Z-Boy and opened the Sunday morning newspaper. I would quickly find the department-store inserts and begin paging through the colored newsprint filled with models

posing in bras and panties. Always smiling. Always available. I loved lingering over each ad insert. It's wrong,
I admitted, but it's such a small thing. It was a far cry
from *Playboy,* I told myself. I peered through the panties,
fantasizing. 📖

8. Which situations in the stories of Steve and Fred can you personally
   identify with most? How common do you think these situations are
   among the Christian men you know?

9. Think about Steve's car wreck for a moment. How much trouble
   have your own eyes gotten you into over the years? What especially
   painful incident stands out to you at the moment?

10. Fred's eyes were particularly vulnerable to the sensual newspaper ads.
    In what situations are your own eyes the most vulnerable? What steps
    have you taken so far to avoid such situations?

11. Recall that, in chapter 3, Fred speaks of the price he was paying for
    his sin in his relationship with God, with his wife, with his children,
    and with his church. In which of these areas of life do you think a
    man's sexual sin hurts him most quickly and obviously? How is it
    with you?

12. In quietness, review what you have written and learned in this week's
    study. If further thoughts or prayer requests come to your mind and
    heart, you may want to write them down.

13. a) What for you was the most meaningful concept or truth in this
       week's study?

    b) How would you talk this over with God? Write your response
       down as a prayer to Him.

    c) What do you believe God wants you to do in response to this
       week's study?

EVERY MAN'S TALK

(Constructive Topics and Questions for Group Discussion)

Key Highlights from the Book for Reading Aloud and Discussing

📖 Addictive sex is devoid of intimacy. Sex addicts are utterly self-focused. They cannot achieve genuine intimacy because their self-obsession leaves no room for giving to others.... Addictive sex is used to escape pain and problems. The escapist nature of addictive sex is often one of the clearest indicators that it is present. 📖

📖 When we're fractionally addicted, we surely experience addictive drawings, but we aren't compelled to act to salve some pain. We're compelled by the chemical high and the sexual gratification it brings. Another way of looking at the scope of the problem is to picture a bell curve. According to our experiences, we figure around 10 percent of men have no sexual-temptation problem with their eyes and their minds. At the other end of the curve, we figure there's another 10 percent of men who are sexual addicts and have a serious problem with lust.... The rest of us comprise the middle 80 percent, living in various shades of gray when it comes to sexual sin. 📖

📖 [From The Heart of a Woman] "When my husband and I talked about this, he was honest," Deena conveyed, "and I was very angry with him. I was hurt. I felt deeply betrayed because I'd been dieting and working out to keep my weight down so that I would always look nice to him.

I couldn't figure out why he still needed to look at other women."

Women told us that they struggle between pity and anger, and their feelings may ebb and flow with the tide of their husband's battle. Let us direct this advice to women reading this book: Though you know you should pray for him and fulfill him sexually, sometimes you won't want to. Talk to each other openly and honestly, then do the right thing. 📖

Discussion Questions

A. Which parts of chapters 1-3 in *Every Man's Battle* were most helpful or encouraging to you and why?

B. How would you summarize the difference between normal sexual desire and addictive sex?

C. Do you agree that sex can be a way of trying to escape inner pain? What is your own experience with this?

D. How would you explain to another man what the authors define as fractional addiction?

E. To what extent do you agree or disagree with the book's contention that, for most men, our sexual sin is based on pleasure-highs rather than true addiction?

F. Look together at The Heart of a Woman quotation. What is most surprising to you in the comments of this woman? What is most helpful to you in better understanding your own wife?

G. Do you agree with the authors' advice to wives? Talk about it together.

H. As an additional group-discussion option, look together at the text under the heading The Heart of a Woman at the end of this week's reading. What is most surprising in the comments of these women? What is most helpful in better understanding your own wife?

how we got here (part A)

This week's reading assignment:

chapters 4–5 in *Every Man's Battle*

For most of us, becoming ensnared by sexual sin happened easily and naturally, like slipping off an icy log.... Perhaps you've mustered the hope that you would someday be free from sexual sin and expected to grow out of it as naturally as you grew into it—like outgrowing acne. Perhaps you waited with each birthday for your sexual impurity to clear up. It never did. Later you assumed you'd be freed naturally through marriage. But—as for many of us—that didn't happen either.

—from chapter 4 in *Every Man's Battle*

📖 EVERY MAN'S TRUTH
(Your Personal Journey into God's Word)

Read and meditate upon the following Bible passages, which deal with God's judgment and mercy—a combination powerfully demonstrated at the Cross of Christ. There, God's *judgment* upon sin *mercifully* freed us from having to experience its destruction. As you study, remember that God's plan is to set sinners free and then use them to teach others.

Be imitators of God, therefore, as dearly loved children
and live a life of love, just as Christ loved us and gave
himself up for us as a fragrant offering and sacrifice
to God.

But among you there must not be even a hint of sexual
immorality, or of any kind of impurity....

For you were once darkness, but now you are light in the
Lord. Live as children of light (for the fruit of the light con-
sists in all goodness, righteousness and truth) and find out
what pleases the Lord. (Ephesians 5:1-3,8-10)

It is God's will that you should be sanctified: that you
should avoid sexual immorality; that each of you should
learn to control his own body in a way that is holy and honorable, not in passionate lust like the heathen, who do not
know God; and that in this matter no one should wrong his
brother or take advantage of him. The Lord will punish men
for all such sins, as we have already told you and warned
you. For God did not call us to be impure, but to live a
holy life. (1 Thessalonians 4:3-7)

Have mercy on me, O God,
    according to your unfailing love;
according to your great compassion
    blot out my transgressions....
Restore to me the joy of your salvation
    and grant me a willing spirit, to sustain me.
Then I will teach transgressors your ways,
    and sinners will turn back to you.
      (Psalm 51:1,12-13)

1. What does Christ's self-sacrifice mean to you? How is it a compelling motive for holy living?

2. What does it mean for you, personally, to live as a child of the light? How can you tell when you're becoming vulnerable to the darkness?

3. How do you respond to the prospect of punishment for sin? In the past, what has been the best motivator, or encourager, to keep you from sexual impurity? What have you been doing to strengthen this motivation in your life?

4. First offer the words of Psalm 51 to God as a heartfelt prayer of your own. Then take a moment to envision how God might use you in the future to minister to another man regarding sexual purity.

☑ EVERY MAN'S CHOICE
(Questions for Personal Reflection and Examination)

📖 When Mark signed up for my premarriage class, he told me, "The whole problem of impurity has been a mess. I've been hooked for years, and I'm counting on marriage to free me. I'll be able to have sex whenever I want it. Satan won't be able to tempt me at all!"

When we got together a few years later, I wasn't surprised to hear that marriage hadn't fixed the problem. Mark said, "You know, Fred…I don't want to seem like a sex addict or anything, but I probably have as many unmet desires now as I did before marriage." 📖

📖 Freedom from sexual sin rarely comes through marriage or the passage of time. (The phrase "dirty old man" should tell us something about that.) So if you're tired of sexual impurity and of the mediocre, distant relationship with God

that results from it, quit waiting for marriage or some hormone drop to save the day. If you want to change, recognize
that you're impure because you've diluted God's standard of
sexual purity with your own. 📖

5. If you were Fred in the conversation above, how would you respond
to Mark?
6. Do you agree that marriage isn't necessarily the "cure" for sexual
impurity? What are the practical implications of this for you?
7. If you've been involved in sexual impurity, how have you experienced
the distant relationship with God referred to by the authors?
8. What kinds of diluting attitudes or actions have you exhibited over
the years?

👟 EVERY MAN'S WALK
(Your Guide to Personal Application)

📖 Sometimes we're simply naive. On his way to school,
Pinocchio met some scoundrels who painted a wonderful
picture of spending the day at a place called Adventure
Island, a sort of amusement park just offshore. He
didn't know that at day's end all the boys would be
turned into donkeys and be sold to pull carts in the
coal mines....

But sometimes we choose wrong sexual standards not
because we're naive, but simply because we're rebellious.
We're like Lampwick, a swaggering boy who takes the lead
in diverting Pinocchio to Adventure Island.... Perhaps, with
a rebelliousness like Lampwick's, you know sexual immorality is wrong, but you do it anyway. You love your trips

to Adventure Island, despite the hidden price you pay at
the end of the day. 📖

📖 It is holy and honorable to completely avoid sexual
immorality—to repent of it, to flee from it, and to put it
to death in our lives, as we live by the Spirit. We've spent
enough time living like pagans in passionate lust. 📖

9. When it comes to succumbing to temptation, would you say you
   are (a) mostly naive, like Pinocchio, or (b) mostly rebellious, like
   Lampwick?

10. What kinds of hidden prices have you paid at the end of a day on
    Adventure Island? (Take a moment to sit quietly with your regret
    and sadness over this. Invite the Lord's presence as you experience
    this pain.)

11. Prayerfully consider: What will it take for me to completely avoid
    sexual immorality in the weeks and years ahead? (Think about any
    changes in your self-image and/or God-image that may be required.
    Also consider what forms of accountability you may need to establish.)

12. In quietness, review what you have written and learned in this week's
    study. If further thoughts or prayer requests come to your mind and
    heart, you may want to write them down.

👥 Every Man's TALK
(Constructive Topics and Questions for Group Discussion)

Key Highlights from the Book for Reading Aloud and Discussing

📖 Sex has different meanings to men and women.
Men primarily receive intimacy just before and during

intercourse. Women gain intimacy through touching, sharing, hugging, and communication. Is it any wonder that the frequency of sex is less important to women than to men? 📖

📖 Larry found Linda to be far more interested in her career than in fulfilling him sexually. Not only was she disinterested in sex, she often used it as a manipulative weapon to get her own way. Consequently, Larry doesn't have sex very often. Twice a month is a bonanza, and once every two months is the norm. What's Larry supposed to say to God? 📖

📖 We aren't victims of some vast conspiracy to ensnare us sexually; we've simply chosen to mix in our own standards of sexual conduct with God's standard. Since we found God's standard too difficult, we created a mixture—something new, something comfortable, something mediocre. 📖

Discussion Questions

A. Which parts of chapter 4 in *Every Man's Battle* were most helpful or encouraging to you and why?

B. Do you agree with the authors' description of how sex has different meanings to men and women? (Optional: How would you add to or modify this statement to make it more relevant to your situation?)

C. Answer the question that comes at the end of Larry's story: What is he supposed to say to God? If you were Larry's best friend, how would you counsel him?

D. If a man has mixed his sexuality standards with God's, what first steps can he take to get back on track? (Brainstorm together about practical actions a man can take, based upon your experience and/or study so far.)

E. In your own words, and in a practical way that would be helpful for Christian men today, how would you summarize God's standards for sexual purity?

Note: If you're following a twelve-week track,
save the rest of this lesson for the following week.
If you're on the eight-week track...then keep going.

☑ EVERY MAN'S CHOICE
(Questions for Personal Reflection and Examination)

📖 Is it profitable for Christians to stop short at the middle ground of excellence where costs are low, balanced somewhere between paganism and obedience? Not at all! While in business it's profitable to seem perfect, in the spiritual realm it's merely comfortable to seem perfect.... Excellence is a mixed standard, while obedience is a fixed standard. We want to shoot for the fixed standard. 📖

📖 If we don't kill every hint of immorality, we'll be captured by our tendency as males to draw sexual gratification and chemical highs through our eyes. But we can't deal with our maleness until we first reject our right to mix standards. As we ask "How holy can I be?" we must pray and commit to a new relationship with God, fully aligned with His call to obedience. 📖

13. How *would* you explain the difference between (a) the pursuit of excellence and (b) the pursuit of perfection (through obedience)?

14. Do you believe you have a right to at least sometimes mix your own standards with God's?

15. Consider the difference in attitude reflected in these two personal questions: (a) How far can I go and still be called a Christian? (b) How holy can I be? How would these attitudes likely manifest themselves in a man's actions?

🥾 EVERY MAN'S WALK
(Your Guide to Personal Application)

📖 God is your Father and expects obedience. Having given you the Holy Spirit as your power source, He believes His command should be enough for you, just as you believe your command should be enough for your kids. Trouble is, we aren't in search of obedience. We're in search of mere excellence, and His command is not enough. We push back, responding, "Why should I eliminate every hint? That's too hard!" 📖

📖 What's your Christian life costing you? It costs something to *learn* about Christ. It costs a lot to *live* like Christ. It costs something to join a few thousand men at a conference to sing praises to God and learn how we should live; it costs a lot to come home and remain committed to the changes you said you'd make in your life.... It costs a lot to control your eyes and mind daily. 📖

16. How would you respond to someone who says: "Why should I eliminate every hint of sexual impurity?"

17. Think through some of the impure temptations and/or practices you've been able to eliminate from your days so far. What hints still remain?

18. Realistically, what is it costing you these days to be a Christian? Try making a list of some of your spiritual price tags. What insight does this list offer?

19. What will likely be the next challenge for you, just over the horizon, when it comes to controlling your eyes and mind? What preparations have you made in order to be ready for the onslaught of temptation?

20. a) What for you was the most meaningful concept or truth in this week's study?

    b) How would you talk this over with God? Write your response down as a prayer to Him.

    c) What do you believe God wants you to do in response to this week's study?

EVERY MAN'S TALK
(More Topics and Questions for Group Discussion)

Key Highlights from the Book for Reading Aloud and Discussing

   Let me demonstrate the difference between excellence and obedience: During transitions between sizes, Brenda often hoped to wear something from her smaller-sized wardrobe to church. Squeezing into it, she'd ask me, "Is this too tight?" Often it was a close call, and I would have to choose between modifying the truth or hurting her feelings and discouraging her. Was it okay for me to modify the truth to avoid this unpleasantness? What would you do? Would you modify the truth? 📖

📖 I organized an intercessors' group during our church's Wednesday night services, simply opening a room for ninety minutes of intercession for our congregation. The first night, a half-dozen people came to the door and asked, "Is this the room where they're teaching about intercession?"

"No, we won't be teaching about intercession," I answered. "We're going to be interceding." Each person turned away to leave. It feels good to learn about intercession, but it's a costly thing to do. The same can be said about purity. 📖

📖 Sexual impurity has become rampant in the church because we've ignored the costly work of obedience to God's standards as individuals, asking too often, "How far can I go and still be called a Christian?" We've crafted an image and may even seem sexually pure while permitting our eyes to play freely when no one is around, avoiding the hard work of being sexually pure. 📖

Discussion Questions

F. Which parts of chapter 5 in *Every Man's Battle* were most helpful or encouraging to you and why?

G. How do you typically answer the question: "Is this dress too tight"? Once the laughter dies down, spend some time in serious discussion about men's tendencies to modify the truth in their approach to sexual purity.

H. Why is it so much easier to learn about prayer than to pray? to learn about purity than to practice purity? What are some of the highest costs involved?

I. Look together at the story of King Josiah in 2 Chronicles 34. Read aloud verse 8 and verses 14-33. How do you see Josiah's example in this passage as a model of obedience? What else is Josiah's example here a model of?

J. When are your eyes most likely to play freely? Talk together about actions or attitudes that help you control your eyes. (Be willing to share what works for you.)

how we got here (part B)

This week's reading assignment:

chapters 6–7 in *Every Man's Battle*

You stand before an important battle. You've decided that the slavery of sexual sin isn't worth your love of sexual sin. You're committed to removing every hint of it. But how? Your maleness looms as your own worse enemy.

You got into this mess by being male; you'll get out by being a man.

—from chapter 7 in *Every Man's Battle*

📖 EVERY MAN'S TRUTH
(Your Personal Journey into God's Word)

As you begin this study, ask for the Holy Spirit's help in hearing and obeying His personal words for you. Read and meditate upon the following Bible passages, which have to do with God's call to faithfulness in marriage. As you read, realize that God is not calling you to anything that's foreign to Himself. The Scriptures proclaim, over and over again, the Lord's utter faithfulness…to *you!*

You shall not commit adultery. (Exodus 20:14)

For these commands are a lamp,

    this teaching is a light,

and the corrections of discipline

    are the way to life,

keeping you from the immoral woman,

    from the smooth tongue of the wayward wife.

Do not lust in your heart after her beauty

    or let her captivate you with her eyes,

for the prostitute reduces you to a loaf of bread,

    and the adulteress preys upon your very life.

Can a man scoop fire into his lap

    without his clothes being burned?

Can a man walk on hot coals

    without his feet being scorched?…

But a man who commits adultery lacks judgment;

    whoever does so destroys himself.

        (Proverbs 6:23-28,32)

He will cover you with his feathers,

    and under his wings you will find refuge;

    his faithfulness will be your shield and rampart.

        (Psalm 91:4)

1. What are some of the horrible consequences of lust and adultery? How does a man destroy himself in the arms of another woman?

2. When you think of God's faithfulness to you, what events or circumstances of the past spring to mind? (Spend some quiet moments in thankfulness and praise.)

3. How does it feel to know that God's love is like the warm and close

protection that a hen offers its young? How can God's faithfulness act as a "shield" and "rampart" in your life?

4. How easy or difficult is it for you, after you have fallen to temptation, to immediately move back under God's "wing"? Why?

☑ EVERY MAN'S **CHOICE**
(Questions for Personal Reflection and Examination)

📖 For males, impurity of the eyes is sexual foreplay. That's right. Just like stroking an inner thigh or rubbing a breast. Because foreplay is any sexual action that naturally takes us down the road to intercourse. Foreplay ignites passions, rocketing us by stages until we go all the way.... No doubt about it: Visual sexual gratification is a form of sex for men. As males, we draw sexual gratification and chemical highs through our eyes. 📖

📖 In a newsletter, author and speaker Dr. Gary Rosberg told of seeing a pair of hands that reminded him of the hands of his father, who had gone on to heaven. Gary continued to reminisce about what his father's hands meant to him. Then he shifted his thoughts to the hands of Jesus, noting this simple truth: "They were hands that never touched a woman with dishonor." 📖

5. Have you ever before considered the dangers of visual foreplay? What is your reaction to the authors' statements about it?

6. What role is visual sexual gratification playing in your life these days? What is your level of awareness of it?

7. Think about the reputation of Jesus' hands for a moment. Then consider: What legacy will your hands leave behind?

8. Read Galatians 6:7-8. How have you seen the truth of this principle in your own life?

EVERY MAN'S WALK
(Your Guide to Personal Application)

    📖 I (Fred) remember the moment when it all broke loose. I'd failed God with my eyes for the thirty-millionth time. My heart churned in guilt, pain, and sorrow. Driving down Merle Hay Road, I suddenly gripped the wheel and through clenched teeth, I yelled out: "That's it! I'm through with this! I'm making a covenant with my eyes. I don't care what it takes, and I don't care if I die trying. It stops here. It stops here!"

    I made that covenant and built it brick by brick. My breakthrough:

- I made a clear decision.
- I decided once and for all to make a change.

    I wasn't fully convinced I could trust myself even then, but I'd finally and truly engaged the battle. Through my covenant with my eyes, all my mental and spiritual resources were now leveled upon a single target: my impurity. With that covenant I had also chosen manhood, to rise above my natural male tendencies. That was a huge step for me. 📖

    📖 Was God proud of Job? You bet! In Job 31:1, we see Job making this startling revelation: "I made a covenant with my eyes not to look lustfully at a girl."

A covenant with his eyes! You mean he made a promise with his eyes to not gaze upon a young woman? It's not possible! It can't be true!

Yet Job was successful; otherwise, he wouldn't have made this promise: "If my heart has been enticed by a woman, or if I have lurked at my neighbor's door, then may my wife grind another man's grain, and may other men sleep with her" (31:9-10). 📖

9. Fred had failed "thirty million" times. How many times has it been for you? Do you believe it will take a crisis-point event like Fred's to bring you to a place of choosing covenant making? Why or why not?

10. Have you ever sensed that the grace of God was the only way out of your cycle of failed will power? How did you respond?

11. What does it mean for you to rest in God's saving grace? How will you know when you are ready to make that your standard response during the toughest temptations?

12. If you were to make a covenant with your eyes right now, how would you write it?

13. In quietness, review what you have written and learned in this week's study. If further thoughts or prayer requests come to your mind and heart, you may want to write them down.

14. a) What for you was the most meaningful concept or truth in this week's study?

b) How would you talk this over with God? Write your response down as a prayer to Him.

c) What do you believe God wants you to do in response to this week's study?

👥 EVERY MAN'S TALK

(Constructive Topics and Questions for Group Discussion)

Key Highlights from the Book for Reading Aloud and Discussing

📖 Author George Gilder in *Sexual Suicide* reported that men commit more than 90 percent of major crimes of violence, 100 percent of the rapes, and 95 percent of the burglaries. Men comprise 94 percent of our drunken drivers, 70 percent of suicides, 91 percent of offenders against family and children. Most often, the chief perpetrators are single men.

Our maleness brings a natural, uniquely male form of rebelliousness. This natural tendency gives us the arrogance needed to stop short of God's standards. As men, we'll often choose sin simply because we like our own way. 📖

📖 "If I'm going to be out all week on business," Rob told us, "Sue and I usually have sex on Sunday night. She's pretty good at helping out that way, and I need the help. On Monday night when I'm on the road, I have dinner, do a little work, catch CNN, and go to bed. I may think about sex, but it's no big deal. By Wednesday night, however, I'm not the same man. I practically feel possessed! The temptations are horrible, and they seem to rise in intensity each night." 📖

📖 When it comes down to it, God's definition of real manhood is pretty simple: It means hearing His Word and doing it. That's God's only definition of manhood—a doer of the Word. And God's definition of a sissy is someone who hears the Word of God and doesn't do it. 📖

Discussion Questions

A. Which parts of chapters 6 and 7 in *Every Man's Battle* were most helpful or encouraging to you and why?

B. Males are rebellious by nature. Obviously this trait is not a gift from God but a result of our sinful nature as fallen human beings. Think about other maleness traits. To what degree is each one a gift from God, and to what degree is each one a result of our sinful nature?

C. To what extent can you relate to Rob's struggles? What is your advice for him?

D. How would you describe the difference between maleness and manhood?

E. Do you totally buy into the conclusion that a real man is one who is a doer of the Word of God? Why or why not?

F. How important is the fellowship of other Christian men when it comes to your ability to be a doer of the Word? What are the opportunities for forming accountability relationships within your group? Talk about it!

G. As an additional group-discussion option, look together at the text under the heading The Heart of a Woman at the end of this week's reading. What is most surprising to you in the comments of these women? What is most helpful to you in better understanding your own wife?

choosing victory (part A)

This week's reading assignment:

chapter 8 in *Every Man's Battle*

When you talk to courageous World War II veterans, they say they don't feel like heroes. They simply had a job to do. When the landing-craft ramps fell open, they swallowed hard and said, "It's time." Time to fight.

In your struggle with sexual impurity, isn't it time? Sure, fighting back will be hard. But your life and home are under a withering barrage of machine-gun sexuality that rakes the landscape mercilessly. Right now you're in a landing craft, inching closer to shore and a showdown. God has given you the weapons and trained you for battle.

You can't stay in the landing craft forever.

—from chapter 8 in *Every Man's Battle*

EVERY MAN'S TRUTH

(Your Personal Journey into God's Word)

As you begin this study, read and meditate upon the following Bible passages, which have to do with your identity and power in Christ. Remember that Christ has already fought the battle against sin on your behalf—and won. Now it is time to live in that victory every day.

Grace and peace be yours in abundance through the knowledge of God and of Jesus our Lord.

His divine power has given us everything we need for life and godliness through our knowledge of him who called us by his own glory and goodness. Through these he has given us his very great and precious promises, so that through them you may participate in the divine nature and escape the corruption in the world caused by evil desires. (2 Peter 1:2-4)

Now if we died with Christ, we believe that we will also live with him. For we know that since Christ was raised from the dead, he cannot die again; death no longer has mastery over him. The death he died, he died to sin once for all; but the life he lives, he lives to God.

In the same way, count yourselves dead to sin but alive to God in Christ Jesus. Therefore do not let sin reign in your mortal body so that you obey its evil desires. Do not offer the parts of your body to sin, as instruments of wickedness, but rather offer yourselves to God, as those who have been brought from death to life; and offer the parts of your body to him as instruments of righteousness. For sin shall not be your master, because you are not under law, but under grace....

You have been set free from sin and have become slaves to righteousness. (Romans 6:8-14,18)

1. According to Peter, what exactly has God given you? What is the source of your ability to "participate in the divine nature"? When

have you most powerfully sensed the glory and goodness of Jesus in your life?

2. If we have everything we need for godliness, what is holding us back from constant, lifelong sexual purity? (Think about what it means to count yourself dead to sin.)

3. In the heat of sexual temptation, what will it mean for you to *not* "offer…your body to sin," as Paul says? What will offering yourself to God require at that point? (Give some thought to the role your will power can play—and *can't* play—at this point in the battle.)

4. Have you ever known someone who was a slave to righteousness? What can you learn from him or her?

☑ EVERY MAN'S CHOICE

(Questions for Personal Reflection and Examination)

📖 I was angry. I wanted to win right away and to win decisively—not somewhere down the road where age might bring victory through the back door. I wanted to win when the battle was hottest.

You should too. If you don't win now, you'll never know whether you're truly a man of God. 📖

📖 We've known those who have failed in their battle for sexual purity, and we know some who have won. The difference? Those who won hated their impurity. They were going to war and were going to win—or die trying. Every resource was leveled upon the foe.

There will be no victory in this area of your life until you choose manhood with all your might. 📖

5. How angry are you about the battle? On a scale of one to ten, how convinced are you that God's will is for you to win the battle and be sexually pure?

6. On a scale of one to ten, to what extent would you say you truly hate the sin of sexual impurity in any form?

7. On a scale of one to ten, to what extent do you truly expect to win the battle for sexual purity? What are your reasons for picking this score?

EVERY MAN'S WALK
(Your Guide to Personal Application)

📖 Listen to the words spoken by preacher Steve Hill, who was addressing escape from addiction to drugs and alcohol as well as from sexual sin: "There's no temptation that is uncommon to man. God will send you a way of escape, but you've got to be willing to take that way of escape, friend." 📖

📖 Admit it: You love your sexual highs, but slavery engulfs you. Is the love worth the loathing?

Look in the mirror. Are you proud of your sexual fantasizing? Or do you feel degraded after viewing lingerie ads or sex scenes in films?

Sexually speaking, you have a low-grade sexual fever. It doesn't disable you, but you aren't healthy either. You can sort of function normally, but you can't really push hard. Basically, you just get by. And if this fever doesn't break, you'll never fully function as a Christian. Like the prodigal son, you need to come to your senses and make a decision. 📖

8. What is your strongest motivation for achieving and maintaining sexual purity?

9. Recall some of the times when you gave in to sexual temptation. Was there always a "way of escape" open to you? In a particular instance, what do you think kept you from taking the escape route?

10. Answer Steve and Fred's question as honestly as you can: "Is the love worth the loathing"? (Suggestion: For a few minutes, turn your awareness to Christ's abiding presence. Just you and Jesus—sit quietly with your response.)

11. Read Romans 12:1-2. Imagine completely giving up sexual fantasy in your life. How much grief would that bring you? Are you ready to experience that pain as an act of sacrificial worship?

12. In quietness, review what you have written and learned in this week's study. If further thoughts or prayer requests come to your mind and heart, you may want to write them down.

13. a) What for you was the most meaningful concept or truth in this week's study?

    b) How would you talk this over with God? Write your response down as a prayer to Him.

    c) What do you believe God wants you to do in response to this week's study?

EVERY MAN'S TALK

(Constructive Topics and Questions for Group Discussion)

Key Highlights from the Book for Reading Aloud and Discussing

📖 Kirk, a worker in a local ministry, was caught in the early stages of an affair. By talking dirty, he'd been pushing a coworker toward a compromising situation. He said he wanted my help, and I (Fred) agreed to meet with Kirk and his pastor.

In our first meeting, the pastor said, "In our community, this kind of talk and behavior is commonplace." I saw Kirk nod his head in agreement. I didn't meet with Kirk again because I knew he didn't hate his sin. 📖

📖 Sexual impurity isn't like a tumor growing out of control inside us. We treat it that way when our prayers focus on deliverance, as we plead for someone to come remove it. Actually, sexual impurity is a series of bad decisions on our part—a result of immature character—and deliverance won't deliver you into instant maturity. Character work needs to be done.

Holiness is not some nebulous thing. It's a series of right choices.... You'll be holy when you choose not to sin. You're already free from the *power* of sexual immorality; you are not yet free from the *habit* of sexual immorality, until you choose to be. 📖

📖 God knows the provision He's made for us. We aren't short on power or authority, but what we lack is urgency. We must choose to be strong and courageous to walk into purity. In the millisecond it takes to make that choice, the Holy Spirit will start guiding you and walking through the struggle with you. 📖

Discussion Questions

A. Which parts of chapter 8 in *Every Man's Battle* were most helpful or encouraging to you and why?

B. Discuss the case of Kirk. Was Fred right in not meeting with him again? Explain.

C. Consider the out-of-control tumor analogy. Why do we tend to think of sexual impurity as a disease that attacks us? How is this a cop-out?

D. What is wrong with praying for deliverance year after year?

E. Describe, as clearly and concisely as you can, the provision God has made for us.

F. Talk in practical terms about what choosing means to you.

G. Take a few moments as a group to reflect silently on these questions as they apply and relate to you: (1) How long are you going to stay sexually impure? (2) How long will you rob your wife sexually? (3) How long will you stunt the growth of oneness with your wife, a oneness you promised her years ago?

choosing victory (part B)

This week's reading assignment:

chapters 9–10 in *Every Man's Battle*

Okay, so you've decided it's time to fight. And you realize that your battle for sexual purity will cost you something. It will require sacrifice, intensity, and honor. But let's get something else in clear view: What can you expect to gain by choosing manhood and the purity that goes with it?

By winning this war, your life will be blessed in tremendous ways. Your victory will recover what was lost through sin. Victory will help you regain and revitalize your relationship with God, your wife, your children, and your ministry.

—from chapter 9 in *Every Man's Battle*

📖 EVERY MAN'S TRUTH
(Your Personal Journey into God's Word)

The following Bible passages continue with the theme of our identity and power in Christ. As you consider their message, ask the Holy Spirit to lead you into specific, practical applications for your daily life.

> Do you not know that your bodies are members of Christ himself? Shall I then take the members of Christ and unite

them with a prostitute? Never! Do you not know that he who unites himself with a prostitute is one with her in body? For it is said, "The two will become one flesh." But he who unites himself with the Lord is one with him in spirit.

Flee from sexual immorality. All other sins a man commits are outside his body, but he who sins sexually sins against his own body. (1 Corinthians 6:15-18)

We take captive every thought to make it obedient to Christ. (2 Corinthians 10:5)

I keep asking that the God of our Lord Jesus Christ, the glorious Father, may give you the Spirit of wisdom and revelation, so that you may know him better. I pray also that the eyes of your heart may be enlightened in order that you may know the hope to which he has called you, the riches of his glorious inheritance in the saints, and his incomparably great power for us who believe. That power is like the working of his mighty strength, which he exerted in Christ when he raised him from the dead and seated him at his right hand in the heavenly realms, far above all rule and authority, power and dominion, and every title that can be given, not only in the present age but also in the one to come. (Ephesians 1:17-21)

1. According to 1 Corinthians 6 above, what is a major implication of being a member of Christ? Have you ever thought of your body as being a part of Christ? What does this mean to you?

2. When are your thoughts typically most "captive"? When are they most likely to roam free?

3. Paul wanted believers to know Jesus better. How can knowing Him

well help us stay sexually pure? How can knowing Him better, day by day, bring power into our lives? (Think about some practical applications to your own battle.)

☑ EVERY MAN'S CHOICE
(Questions for Personal Reflection and Examination)

📖 Because of sin, I (Fred) hadn't been able to look at myself in a mirror for years. While I knew God loved me unconditionally, I also knew He didn't unconditionally approve of my behavior. Consequently, I couldn't look God in the eye.

Once I heard a pastor preach, "When Jesus knocks, He wants freedom to enter every room in your house. In every part of your life, He wants to be welcome and comfortable. Is He locked out of any room in your house?" 📖

📖 I (Fred) was a prodigal eating old cobs of corn left in a pigsty. To restore my relationship with my Father, I had to get up out of the mud and start walking home. I didn't have to clean myself up first, but I did have to make that first step. On the road ahead, the Father would be waiting with a ring, a robe, shoes, and everything else an honored son was meant to have. But first I had to come to my senses, as I did that day on Merle Hay Road when I took my first step toward home—toward purity—by making that covenant with my eyes. 📖

4. Can you look at yourself in the mirror these days? Can you look God in the eye? Think about it…

5. Make a list of the rooms in your inner "house" where Jesus is welcome and unwelcome. What keeps certain rooms off-limits to Him, even though He already knows what's there? (Suggestion: Spend some moments, right now, letting Jesus into the ugliest rooms. Tell Him of the longing, desire, pain, and so on, that has helped you "furnish" those rooms over the years. This is an opportunity to open your whole heart to Him.)

6. If you see some aspects of the prodigal son within you, where are you in your journey? Are you still heading for adventure in the big, wide world? suffering loss and desperation? on your way back home?

EVERY MAN'S **WALK**
(Your Guide to Personal Application)

> One of the things I (Steve) brought into my marriage with Sandy was a secret compartment I'd guarded for years. Inside it was a girlfriend from much earlier in my life, the first true love I really had. I considered this secret compartment to be mine forever, a private place out of which I could draw fond old memories. It wasn't until I was willing to give up that secret compartment that I was fully able to connect with Sandy.

> Likewise, sin can affect families for generations, as it did in mine. I came from a family in which the men loved sex and pornography and ditched their wives or were caught up in affairs....
>
> My sixteen-year-old son, Jasen, is now a handsome, strapping, six-foot adolescent with an easy smile and friendly ways. Not long ago Jasen was with friends who had some

pornography. He walked away. My son walked away. You don't understand what that means to me! 📖

7. To what extent can you relate to Steve's secret compartment? Do you have any compartments labeled Old Girlfriends or Pornography or Favorite Web Sites? What practical steps can you take—today—to begin forsaking these private, secret compartments?

8. How have you been affected by the sins of your fathers? How do you think you are affecting your own children's lives through your secret sins of impurity?

9. Be Fred for a moment. How do you feel after discovering that Jasen walked away from pornography? Would your son (or any child who looks to your example) walk away?

10. As you think of attaining the sexual purity that is God's will for you, how do you envision your relationship with God in the near future? your relationship with your wife? your future legacy for your children? your ministry in the church, both in the near future and long-term?

11. In quietness, review what you have written and learned in this week's study. If further thoughts or prayer requests come to your mind and heart, you may want to write them down.

👥 EVERY MAN'S TALK

(Constructive Topics and Questions for Group Discussion)

Key Highlights from the Book for Reading Aloud and Discussing

📖 Along with inner peace comes an outer peace that affects your daily life.... Wally used to dread hotels. He can now check into a hotel at night, enjoy a meal at the coffee shop, go back to his room, shower, turn out the lights, and fall asleep. "I no longer fear hotel rooms in the slightest," he says. "Sensual things don't dominate my day as they once could. All those compelling desires that ruled me are gone, and yet my desire for my wife, Tina, still percolates rather nicely!" 📖

📖 Trust is important in the body of Christ. In 1 Corinthians 6:15-20, Paul says that not only does a sexually immoral man sin against his own body, but he also sins against the body of Christ and his friends within the body. Our friends trust us to be pure; a failure would crush their spirits as well as our own. We must be trustworthy. 📖

📖 When your son questions what he should watch, what he should do with the pornography other boys show him, or what he should do when that cute girl gets him alone and starts unbuttoning her blouse, will anyone be speaking against it? It won't be his friends. Even his church buddies will tell him to go for it. Your voice had better be loud and crystal clear because it will probably be the only one whispering, "Flee immorality, son." Your example must be the argument opposing temptation. 📖

Discussion Questions

A. Which parts of chapter 9 in *Every Man's Battle* were most helpful or encouraging to you and why?

B. Talk about Wally and the change that occurred in his life. In your opinion, how realistic is it to think that any man could come to this point— of not being tempted by the X-rated cable channels in the motel room?

C. Talk together about the trust levels in your group, in light of the middle quotation above. Discuss some ways you can maintain trust with one another in the area of sexual purity.

D. Look at the last quotation on the previous page. Sit for a while in silence as each man does a personal example check within his heart. Then spend some time praying for one another's children and/or the young men in your church or community.

Note: If you're following a twelve-week track,
save the rest of this lesson for the following week.
If you're on the eight-week track...then keep going.

☑ EVERY MAN'S CHOICE
(Questions for Personal Reflection and Examination)

📖 Satan's greatest weapon against you is deception. He knows Jesus has already purchased your freedom. He also knows that once you see the simplicity of this battle, you'll win in short order, so he deceives and confuses. He tricks you into thinking you're a helpless victim, someone who'll need years of group therapy. 📖

📖 Your goal is sexual purity. Here's a good working definition of it—good because of its simplicity: You are sexually pure when no sexual gratification comes from anyone or anything but your wife.

Purity means stopping sexual gratification that comes to us from outside our marriage.... That means your objective in the war against lust is to build three perimeters of defense into your life: (1) with your eyes, (2) in your mind, and (3) in your heart. 📖

12. Have you ever viewed yourself as a helpless victim to sexual temptation? According to Steve and Fred, what is a more honest assessment?

13. What is your reaction to the authors' definition of sexual purity? To what extent are you ready to put it into daily practice?

👟 EVERY MAN'S WALK
(Your Guide to Personal Application)

📖 The simple truth? Impurity is a habit. It lives like a habit. When some hot-looking babe walks in, your eyes have the bad habit of bouncing toward her, sliding up and down.... The fact that impurity is merely a habit comes as a surprise to many men.... If impurity were genetic or some victimizing spell, you'd be helpless. But since impurity is a habit, it can be changed. You have hope, because if it lives like a habit, it can die like a habit. (We believe it can be done in six weeks.) 📖

📖 Don't misunderstand. We're not saying your habits have no relationship to your emotions or circumstances. Glen told us, "My sexual sin became much worse when I was under a deadline at work, and especially when my wife and I fought or I felt unloved and unappreciated. It seemed at those times that I was compelled to sin sexually and couldn't say no."

For Glen, job-related stress and lack of acceptance were *not* the root cause of his sexual impurity, however. The

sexual impurity was simply one way he dealt with these
emotions and circumstances. In short, he ran to impurity
as an escape. But when he removed the sexual impurity,
he began processing these things in other ways. 📖

14. Consider why the authors believe impurity and masturbation are
    habits. To what extent do you agree or disagree with their reasoning?

15. Think of some habits that you've "killed" in the past. Do you believe
    the impurity habit can die as well? What gives you hope?

16. Glen experienced an increased compulsion during times of stress,
    anger, or rejection. Can you relate? What could help you prepare for
    these times of particular vulnerability in the future?

17. a) What for you was the most meaningful concept or truth in this
       week's study?

    b) How would you talk this over with God? Write your response
       down as a prayer to Him.

    c) What do you believe God wants you to do in response to this
       week's study?

😊😊 EVERY MAN'S TALK

(More Topics and Questions for Group Discussion)

Key Highlights from the Book for Reading Aloud and Discussing

📖 Because of rejection and lost love, men begin to seek for
this lost love in all the wrong places. In their search, where's
the path of least resistance? A pretend lover, a pornographic
lover with a permanent smile. A lover who never says no, one
who never rejects. One who never abandons and is always discreet. One who supports the man's ego in the midst of his

self-doubt.... This path is a *chosen* path, a path made available by the impure eyes stoking the sexual fever, providing an unending pool of lovers from which to draw. 📖

📖 While there may not be spiritual oppression involved in your battle, there'll always be spiritual opposition. The enemy is constantly near your ear. He doesn't want you to win this fight, and he knows the lies that so often break men's confidence and their will to win. Expect to hear lies and plenty of them. 📖

📖 The first issue is accountability. For many men who are willing to fight for sexual purity, an important step is finding accountability support in a men's Bible study group, in a smaller group of one or two other men serving as accountability partners, or by going into counseling.

For an accountability partner, enlist a male friend, perhaps someone older and well respected in the church, to encourage you in the heat of battle. The men's ministry at your church can also help you find someone who can pray for you and ask you the tough questions. 📖

Discussion Questions

E. Which parts of chapter 10 in *Every Man's Battle* were most helpful or encouraging to you and why?

F. What is the authors' working definition of sexual purity in this chapter? What are the three defense perimeters they say we must build to attain the goal of sexual purity?

G. The authors say: "Expect to hear lies and plenty of them." Look at Satan's arguments listed under the heading Purity Always Brings Spiritual Opposition. Which of these arguments do you think are the most powerful and dangerous? Which of the truth-responses are most encouraging to you?

H. What is your experience with seeking love in the wrong places? Do you agree this has been a choice? How does rejection or lost love tend to fuel this choice?

I. Have someone read aloud the third quote above, dealing with accountability. Then go back to the conversation in the book between Ron and Nathan. As appropriate, talk together about how these kinds of relationships could work among some of the men in your group. Do any of the men want to set up an accountability relationship at this time?

J. As an additional group-discussion option, look together at the text under the heading The Heart of a Woman at the end of this week's reading. What is most surprising to you in the comments of these women? What is most helpful to you in better understanding your own wife?

victory with your eyes

This week's reading assignment:
chapters 11-13 in *Every Man's Battle*

Why must "bouncing the eyes" be immediate? After all, you might argue, a glance isn't the same as lusting. If we define "lusting" as staring open-mouthed until drool pools at your feet, then a glance isn't the same as lusting. But if we define lusting as any look that creates that little chemical high, that little pop, then we have something a bit more difficult to measure. This chemical high happens more quickly than you realize. In our experience, drawing the line at "immediate" is clean and easy for the mind and eyes to understand.

—adapted from chapter 11 in *Every Man's Battle*

EVERY MAN's TRUTH
(Your Personal Journey into God's Word)

Read and meditate upon the following Bible passages, which have to do with the marvelous visual aspects of God's creation. Let the Lord bless you as you remember: He gave you sight that you might enjoy all the beauty and wonder of this world. The ultimate goal, of course, is that your heart may be lifted up in praise of His awesome power and glory. Why let your eyes pursue less worthy goals?

O LORD, our Lord,

how majestic is your name in all the earth!

You have set your glory

above the heavens....

When I consider your heavens,

the work of your fingers,

the moon and the stars,

which you have set in place,

what is man that you are mindful of him,

the son of man that you care for him?

(Psalm 8:1,3-4)

The heavens declare the glory of God;

the skies proclaim the work of his hands.

Day after day they pour forth speech;

night after night they display knowledge.

There is no speech or language

where their voice is not heard.

(Psalm 19:1-3)

My eyes are ever on the LORD,

for only he will release my feet from the snare.

(Psalm 25:15)

1. Consider the majesty of God conveyed by the heavens. When have you experienced this awesomeness in a night sky? Give thanks!

2. How can creation "display knowledge"? What have you seen of God in nature?

3. If you've been using your eyes more for lust than for worship, what would you like to say to the Lord about that right now? Consider:

What practical actions might help you to keep your eyes "ever on the Lord" this day?

☑ EVERY MAN'S CHOICE
(Questions for Personal Reflection and Examination)

📖 A red-blooded American male can't watch a major sporting event without being assaulted by commercials showing a bunch of half-naked women cavorting on some beach with some beer-soaked yahoos. What's a man to do? 📖

📖 To attain sexual purity as we defined it, we must starve our eyes of the bowls of sexual gratification that come from outside our marriage. When you starve your eyes and eliminate "junk sex" from your life, you'll deeply crave "real food"—your wife. And no wonder. She's the only thing in the cupboard, and you're hungry! 📖

4. Think about the red-blooded American male's dilemma in front of the television. What is Fred's solution? Define "bouncing the eyes."

5. How many bowls of gratification do you think you receive from "junk sex" in a typical day? What will starving the eyes look like or you? And are you ready to crave your wife more deeply?

👟 EVERY MAN'S WALK
(Your Guide to Personal Application)

📖 I (Fred) can't define the best defense for your weaknesses, but let me share mine so you'll get a feel for the process.

Rule 1: When my hand reached for a magazine or insert, if I sensed in even the slightest way that my underlying motive was to see something sensual, I forfeited my right to pick up that magazine or insert. Forever.

To be honest, this didn't work well at first. 📖

📖 My body began to fight back in some interesting ways....

Whenever I was taken in by one of these tricks, I'd bark to myself in sharp rebuke, "You've made a covenant with your eyes! You can't do that anymore." In the first two weeks, I must have said it a million times, but the repeated confession of truth eventually worked a transformation in me. 📖

6. Look over Fred's list of My Greatest Enemies in chapter 11. What would be on your own list of "obvious and prolific sources of sensual images apart from your wife"? (Spend plenty of time coming up with an accurate list that doesn't overlook any important areas.)

7. Now spend plenty of time coming up with defense tactics in each identified area.

8. Fred says he can't define the actual defense methods that will work best for you. But what did you think of his own rules? What about rule number one? What rules are you considering for yourself?

9. Are you ready for your body and mind to fight back, as Fred's did? What forms of inner rebellion will you likely need to prepare yourself for in this battle?

10. In quietness, review what you have written and learned in this week's study. If further thoughts or prayer requests come to your mind and heart, you may want to write them down.

👥 EVERY MAN'S TALK

(Constructive Topics and Questions for Group Discussion)

Key Highlights from the Book for Reading Aloud and Discussing

📖 Imagine that your current level of sexual hunger requires ten bowls of sexual gratification per week. These bowls of gratification should be filled from your single legitimate vessel, the wife whom God provided for you. But because males soak up sexual gratification through the eyes, we can effortlessly fill our bowls from other sources. 📖

📖 Once you're winning the battle, you'll be saying things you haven't uttered for years like, "I can't wait for tonight, baby." All your imaginative creativity now blossoms upon your marriage bed, not in some fantasy world. You'll be fully enamored with her!... She'll probably ask you what's going on, and once she learns what's cooking, you'll both need to find a new sexual equilibrium. 📖

📖 "Wait a minute, Fred," you say. "Cutting down from ten bowls to eight bowls seems unfair. I'm being cheated, all because I'm obeying God!"

I guarantee you won't feel cheated. With your whole sexual being now focused upon your wife, sex with her will be so transformed that your satisfaction will explode off any known scale. Yes, even while consuming fewer bowls. It's a personal guarantee.... You can count on a sexual payoff from obedience. 📖

Discussion Questions

A. Which parts of chapters 11 and 12 in *Every Man's Battle* were most helpful or encouraging to you and why?

B. What is your reaction to the bowls analogy? How helpful is it for you to view your sexual need this way? Why?

C. How do you think most wives will respond to a husband who's newly enamored with her? How would you counsel a friend in this situation, as he helps his wife learn what's going on?

D. In your opinion, what percentage of men will likely react to starving the eyes with: "I'm being cheated"? Why? What is the authors' response?

Note: If you're following a twelve-week track,
save the rest of this lesson for the following week.
If you're on the eight-week track...then keep going.

☑ EVERY MAN'S CHOICE
(Questions for Personal Reflection and Examination)

📖 You'll need a good Bible verse to use as a sword and rallying point.... But your shield—a protective verse that you can reflect on and draw strength from even when you aren't in the direct heat of battle—may be even more important than your sword, because it places temptation out of earshot. 📖

11. Why do you need a "sword" and "shield," according to this chapter? What is their value in your pursuit of sexual purity?

12. What are the merits of Job 31:1 as a "sword" verse? As a challenge to this verse, what thoughts or arguments do you think Satan and his forces would be likely to use?

13. What are the merits of 1 Corinthians 6:18-20 as a "shield" passage? As a challenge to this passage, what thoughts or arguments do you think Satan and his forces would be likely to use?

14. What aspects of the authors' strategy for bouncing and starving the eyes make the most sense to you? What questions do you still have about these plans?

EVERY MAN'S WALK
(Your Guide to Personal Application)

Suddenly an old girlfriend pops into your mind. Note the great difference in perspective between the following two possible responses:

1. Should I daydream about my old girlfriend right now?

2. I don't even have the right to ask such a question, because I don't have the authority to make that decision.

The first response implies that you have the authority and the right to make that decision. The second implies that the question itself is moot.

In the long term, do you still have to monitor your eyes? Yes, because the natural bent of your eyes is to sin, and you'll return to bad habits if you're careless. But with only the slightest effort, good habits are permanent....

After a year or so—though it may take longer—nearly all major skirmishes will stop. Bouncing your eyes will become deeply entrenched. Your brain, now policing itself tightly, will

rarely slip anymore, having given up long ago on its chances
to return to the old days of pornographic pleasure-highs. 📖

15. What verses will you select for your "sword" and for your "shield"?

16. What are some of the important questions in the realm of sexual
temptation that you no longer have a right to ask yourself?

17. What kind of short-term results and reactions do you expect in your
pursuit of sexual purity? What kind of long-term results and reactions
do you expect in your pursuit of sexual purity?

18. In your own life, what do you believe are the most important factors
that will ensure the success of this entire strategy for purity through
your eyes?

19. a) What for you was the most meaningful concept or truth in this
week's study?

b) How would you talk this over with God? Write your response
down as a prayer to Him.

c) What do you believe God wants you to do in response to this
week's study?

👥 EVERY MAN'S TALK

(More Topics and Questions for Group Discussion)

Key Highlights from the Book for Reading Aloud and Discussing

📖 Once on an overnight hotel stay, I walked down the
hallway to the ice machine. On top of the machine was a
Playboy magazine. Believing I had a right to choose my
behavior, I asked myself this question: Should I look at this
Playboy or not?

The moment I asked that question, I opened myself to counsel. I began talking pros and cons to myself. But far worse, I opened myself to Satan's counsel. He wanted to be heard on this issue....

Therein lies the power of temptation. You may fear that temptation will be too strong for you in this battle, but temptations honestly have no power at all without our own arrogant questions. 📖

📖 Looking back at the details of our plan, even we will admit that it all sounds slightly crazy. Defenses, brain tricks, bouncing your eyes, forfeiting rights. Man! We wonder if even Job would be a bit startled.

On the other hand, maybe we should expect a sound plan to look this way. Consider all the men who are called to purity, yet so few seem to know how to do it. 📖

Discussion Questions

E. Which parts of chapter 13 in *Every Man's Battle* were most helpful or encouraging to you and why?

F. Have you ever "been there" at the ice machine with Fred? What did you do in a similar situation?

G. According to Fred, what is the problem with getting into a conversation with ourselves about how we should respond to a particular temptation?

H. Fred and Steve admit that their plan for purity may seem slightly crazy. Have you had that reaction during this course of study? Talk about it!

I. As an additional group-discussion option, look together at the text under the heading The Heart of a Woman at the end of this week's reading. What is most surprising to you in the comments of these women? What is most helpful to you in better understanding your own wife?

victory with your mind

This week's reading assignment:
chapters 14-16 in *Every Man's Battle*

The great news is that the defense perimeter of the eyes works with you to build the perimeter of the mind. The mind needs an object for its lust, so when the eyes view sexual images, the mind has plenty to dance with. Without those images, the mind has an empty dance card. By starving the eyes, you starve the mind as well.

—from chapter 14 in *Every Man's Battle*

EVERY MAN'S TRUTH
(Your Personal Journey into God's Word)

As you begin this week's study, read and meditate upon the following Bible passages, which deal with appreciating God's grace, love, and power. Remember that you can choose to fill your mind with thoughts of God's goodness throughout your day. Think on these things!

> Answer me, O LORD, out of the goodness of your love;
>> in your great mercy turn to me.
> Do not hide your face from your servant;
>> answer me quickly, for I am in trouble.

Come near and rescue me;

redeem me because of my foes.

(Psalm 69:16-18)

Praise be to the God and Father of our Lord Jesus Christ, who has blessed us in the heavenly realms with every spiritual blessing in Christ. For he chose us in him before the creation of the world to be holy and blameless in his sight. In love he predestined us to be adopted as his sons through Jesus Christ, in accordance with his pleasure and will—to the praise of his glorious grace, which he has freely given us in the One he loves. In him we have redemption through his blood, the forgiveness of sins, in accordance with the riches of God's grace that he lavished on us with all wisdom and understanding. (Ephesians 1:3-8)

Finally, brothers, whatever is true, whatever is noble, whatever is right, whatever is pure, whatever is lovely, whatever is admirable—if anything is excellent or praiseworthy—think about such things. (Philippians 4:8)

1. Have you ever prayed the words of Psalm 69 that King David prayed? Do you have this fellow sinner's confidence in God's goodness, love, and mercy?

2. Meditate upon the blessings proclaimed in Ephesians 1:3-8. Make a list of the spiritual riches bestowed upon you as an adopted son of the heavenly Father. How will you live as His son today?

3. To what extent will your mind need transforming if you are to carry out the apostle's command in Philippians 4:8?

☑ EVERY MAN'S CHOICE

(Questions for Personal Reflection and Examination)

📖 Your mind is orderly, and your worldview colors what comes through it. The mind will allow impure thoughts only if they "fit" the way you look at the world. As you set up the perimeter of defense for your mind, your brain's worldview will be transformed by a new matrix of allowed thoughts, or "allowables."…

This transformation of the mind takes some time as you wait for the old sexual pollution to be washed away. It's much like living near a creek that becomes polluted when a sewer main breaks upstream. After repair crews replace the cracked sewage pipe, it will still take some time for the water downstream to clear. 📖

📖 Have you "lurked at your neighbor's door"? It could mean stopping by in the late afternoon, visiting your friend's wife for coffee, enamored by her wisdom, care, and sensitivity. You felt sorry for her as you've commiserated together over her insensitive, brutish husband. You held her as she cried. You were lurking at your neighbor's door. 📖

4. Why is the mind more difficult to control than the eyes? How will your eyes work together with your mind in your pursuit of sexual purity?
5. What do the authors mean by "lurking at the door" and "mental lurking"? What is your own experience with this?

👟 EVERY MAN'S WALK

(Your Guide to Personal Application)

📖 According to Jesus, doing it mentally is the same as doing it physically. 📖

📖 Currently, your mind runs like a mustang. What's more, your mind "mates" where it wills with attractive, sensual women. They're everywhere. With a mustang mind, how do you stop the running and the mating? With a corral around your mind. 📖

6. How seriously do you take Jesus' words in Matthew 5:28?
7. How would you explain the authors' corral concept as it applies to sexual purity in your thought life? What does the corral represent, and what does it accomplish?
8. How useful do you think this corral concept can be for you?
9. In quietness, review what you have written and learned in this week's study. If further thoughts or prayer requests come to your mind and heart, you may want to write them down.

👥 EVERY MAN'S TALK

(Constructive Topics and Questions for Group Discussion)

Key Highlights from the Book for Reading Aloud and Discussing

📖 The defense perimeter of the mind is less like a wall and more like a customs area in an international airport. Customs departments are filters, preventing dangerous elements from entering a country. The U.S. Customs Service

attempts to filter out drugs, Mediterranean fruit flies, terrorists, and other harmful agents.

Similarly, the defense perimeter of the mind properly
processes attractive women into your "country," filtering out
the alien seeds of attraction before the impure thoughts are
even generated. This perimeter "stops the lurking." 📖

📖 Jack: "I knew that kiss would end my career at my
church, but I couldn't help myself." 📖

Discussion Questions

A. Which parts of chapter 14 in *Every Man's Battle* were most helpful or
   encouraging to you and why?
B. How would you explain the process, as explained in this chapter, by
   which the mind cleans away old sexual pollution? What encouragement does understanding this process give you?
C. What do the authors mean by a "mental customs station"? Describe
   this process in practical terms.
D. What do the authors mean by "starving the attractions"? What would
   it mean practically in your life?
E. Recall Fred's story of his high-school crush on Judy—and the disaster
   prom date that ended it. Fred said: "My attractions to Judy died that
   night. The facts did them in!" Discuss the problem of filling in the
   blanks versus letting the facts do their attraction-reducing work.

Note: If you're following a twelve-week track,

save the rest of this lesson for the following week.

If you're on the eight-week track…then keep going.

☑ EVERY MAN'S **CHOICE**
(Questions for Personal Reflection and Examination)

📖 Think about two types of women who will approach your corral:
- Women you find attractive;
- Women who find you attractive.

Both categories have similar defenses, each designed to starve the attractions until she trots off toward the horizon. 📖

10. What are the most important principles for having effective defenses against impure thoughts regarding women you find attractive?
11. What are the most important principles for having effective defenses against impure thoughts regarding women who find you attractive?
12. What is your level of temptation toward old girlfriends and/or ex-wives? wives of friends? What are the authors' most helpful suggestions to you in these areas?

👟 EVERY MAN'S **WALK**
(Your Guide to Personal Application)

📖 Always play the dweeb. Players flirt.... Learn to un-flirt. Players banter.... Learn to un-banter. If a woman smiles with a knowing look, learn to smile with a slightly confused look, to un-smile. If she talks about things that are hip, talk about things that are un-hip to her, like your wife and kids. She'll find you pleasant enough but rather bland and uninteresting. Perfect. 📖

📖 It's not that you don't trust your friend's wife; it's that you don't want to start anything. She should be like a sister to you, with no hint of attraction between you.

You'll always have some relationship with your friend's wife, but limit it to when your friend is around. This isn't always possible, but some simple rules can shield you from surprise attacks within the corral. 📖

13. Review the four "shields" from surprise attacks related to friends' wives. Consider the practicality of each suggestion for your own life.

14. What do the authors mean by "playing the dweeb," and how effective do you think this tactic can be in your own life?

15. In your own life, what do you believe are the most important factors that will ensure the success of the authors' entire strategy for purity (that is, bouncing, starving, corralling, playing the dweeb, and so on)?

16. a) What for you was the most meaningful concept or truth in this week's study?

b) How would you talk this over with God? Write your response down as a prayer to Him.

c) What do you believe God wants you to do in response to this week's study?

😊😊 EVERY MAN'S TALK

(More Topics and Questions for Group Discussion)

Key Highlights from the Book for Reading Aloud and Discussing

📖 For those women who are already within your corral, the situation becomes rather complicated. These women won't drift back to the horizon. They're in your corral today and probably will be there tomorrow and the next day. This means you must eliminate these attractions in some other way. Let's take a look at the two main categories of women within your corral: old girlfriends and ex-wives; wives of your friends. 📖

📖 In *The Final Quest,* Rick Joyner writes, "Spiritual maturity is always dictated by our willingness to sacrifice our own desires for the desires of others or for the interests of the kingdom."

Purifying your eyes and mind is more than a command—it's also a sacrifice. And as you make that sacrifice, as you lay down your desires, blessings will flow. Your spiritual life will experience new joy and power, and your marriage life will blossom as your relationship reaches new heights. 📖

Discussion Questions

F. Which parts of chapters 15 and 16 in *Every Man's Battle* were most helpful or encouraging to you and why?

G. What tactics were presented for maintaining pure thoughts in regard to old girlfriends and ex-wives? What is your opinion of their effectiveness?

H. What tactics were presented for maintaining pure thoughts in regard to the wives of your friends? Why is it important to think through this strategy? (Spend several minutes talking about the practical implications for your group.)

I. As an additional group-discussion option, look together at the text under the heading The Heart of a Woman at the end of this week's reading. What is most surprising to you in the comments of these women? What is most helpful to you in better understanding your own wife?

victory in your heart

This week's reading assignment:

chapters 17-18 in *Every Man's Battle*

Let's talk about your innermost perimeter, which is about being consumed with God's purpose to cherish your wife. If Christians were consumed by God's purposes, it would first be reflected in our marriages. But the rates of divorce, adultery, and marital dissatisfaction in the Christian church reveal our hearts. We've known very few men consumed by their marriages, and fewer still consumed by purity, but both are God's desire for you. God's purpose for your marriage is that it parallels Christ's relationship to His church, that you be one with your wife.

—from chapter 17 in *Every Man's Battle*

📖 EVERY MAN'S TRUTH

(Your Personal Journey into God's Word)

As you begin this final study, take some time to read and meditate upon the following Bible passage, which has to do with the beauty of the bride—the bride of Christ and also your own bride. Keep in mind that, for centuries, the Song of Solomon has often been viewed as an allegory of how Christ feels for His bride (all believers).

> How beautiful you are, my darling!
>> Oh, how beautiful!
>> Your eyes behind your veil are doves....
> Your lips are like a scarlet ribbon;
>> Your mouth is lovely....
> All beautiful you are, my darling;
>> there is no flaw in you....
> You have stolen my heart, my sister, my bride;
>> you have stolen my heart
> with one glance of your eyes....
> How delightful is your love, my sister, my bride!...
> Your head crowns you like Mount Carmel.
>> Your hair is like royal tapestry;
>> the king is held captive by its tresses.
> How beautiful you are and how pleasing,
>> O love, with your delights!
>>> (Song of Songs 4:1,3,7,9-10; 7:5-6)

1. Do you sense Jesus' desire for you as part of His bride? In return, does your heart yearn for Him like this?
2. Because our marriage relationships should parallel Christ's relationship to the church, our feelings for our wives should parallel these passages. Can you be content with the wife of your youth? (If she isn't all you'd hoped for, remember that God graced you with this ewe lamb.)
3. Can you make a commitment to cherish her today?

☑ EVERY MAN'S CHOICE

(Questions for Personal Reflection and Examination)

> 📖 Are you cherishing your wife? Do you feel
> cherished?
>
> If not, you probably got there the same way I did—
> by stopping short of God's standards. God's standard
> is to unconditionally cherish her, no matter what.
> No conditions. But in America, we've added mealy-
> mouthed terms to form "conditional contracts."…
> The problem comes when we expect our wives to
> deliver these things under contractual conditions.
> With Brenda, anger and resentment erupted when
> I felt she didn't carry her side of the bargain. I no
> longer felt like cherishing her. 📖

4. Review carefully the teaching in Ephesians 5:25-33 in light of all you've learned in this book and your study during the previous weeks. Why do you think so many husbands tend to resist the teaching of this passage?

5. State in your own words what the passage above teaches in regard to your marriage and Christ's relationship to the church. What are the right attitudes and convictions as taught in this passage? What are the right standards and ideals? What are the right actions and habits?

6. What does it really mean to you to cherish your wife?

7. What contractual conditions have you been trying to hold your wife to over the years? Were you consciously aware of doing this? What now needs to change?

👟 EVERY MAN'S WALK
(Your Guide to Personal Application)

📖 Your wife gave up her freedom for you. She relinquished her rights to seek happiness elsewhere. She exchanged this freedom for something she considered more valuable: your love and your word. Her dreams are tied up in you, dreams of sharing and communication and oneness.

She's pledged to be yours sexually. Her sexuality is her most guarded possession, her secret garden. She trusted you would be worthy of this gift, but you have cavalierly viewed sensual garbage, polluting and littering her garden. She deserves more, and you must honor that. 📖

📖 In my office I keep an eight-by-ten, black-and-white photo of Brenda when she was one year old. Her little eyes sparkle and are filled with the hope and joy of life, her mischievous smile apparent even then; her glowing, chubby cheeks radiating joy and a carefree spirit. That face is so full of expectations and wonder. I brought that infant picture to my office because it reminds me that I need to honor that hope. 📖

8. What has your wife given up for you? What are the most important things your wife has given to you?

9. What are the most important honor issues in your marriage? What are the most important ways you can build up and honor your wife's hope?

10. What can you do today to more faithfully honor your wife? What can you do tomorrow? What can you do as a new habit for the rest of your life together?

11. In quietness, review what you have written and learned in this week's study. If further thoughts or prayer requests come to your mind and heart, you may want to write them down.

12. a) What for you was the most meaningful concept or truth in this week's study?

b) How would you talk this over with God? Write your response down as a prayer to Him.

c) What do you believe God wants you to do in response to this week's study?

👥 EVERY MAN'S TALK
(Constructive Topics and Questions for Group Discussion)

Key Highlights from the Book for Reading Aloud and Discussing

> 📖 What does the standard of Christ's relationship to His church have to do with our sexual purity? In our hearts, we often have selfish attitudes and expectations regarding our wives. When these expectations aren't met, we become grumpy and frustrated. Our will to maintain our outer defense perimeters is eroded. Well, if this is how she's going to be, why should I go through all the effort of being pure? She doesn't deserve it. We retaliate by withdrawing from our own responsibilities. 📖

> 📖 Uriah knew his place. He was satisfied to be part of God's purposes, to fill his role. To be like Uriah, we must know our place and be content with it. 📖

📖 In our society, we have "sensitivity training" and "cross-cultural enrichment" classes. We believe if we can only teach people the "right" feelings, they'll act correctly. In the Bible, however, God tells us the opposite: We're to first act correctly, and then right feelings will follow.

If you don't feel like cherishing, cherish anyway. Your right feelings will arrive soon enough. 📖

Discussion Questions

A. Which parts of chapters 17 and 18 in *Every Man's Battle* were most helpful or encouraging to you and why?

B. When have you been grumpy and frustrated when your expectations for your wife haven't been met? Can you share about a recent example? How do you typically retaliate for unmet expectations?

C. Under the heading How Cherishing Feels in chapter 17, look at the authors' paraphrases from the Song of Solomon. How would you analyze the feelings conveyed in these passages? How helpful are these passages as tools for understanding your proper emotional involvement with your wife?

D. Look at the quotation above about Uriah and then review the story of David, Bathsheba, Uriah, and Nathan (from 2 Samuel 11–12) as summarized by the authors. This is probably a story you've read before. As you consider it again, what stands out to you, now that you've carefully studied sexual purity and made a commitment to pursue it? What are the most important lessons this story has for Christian men today in their marriages?

E. Do you agree that we're to first act correctly and then right feelings will follow? Why or why not? What is your evidence?

F. Take a moment to reflect on what you've studied and discussed during the previous weeks. Ask each man to comment on one or more of these questions:

1. What can you thank God for as a result of this study?

2. What do you sense that God most wants you to understand at this time about this topic?

3. In what specific ways do you believe He wants you now to more fully trust and obey Him?

don't keep it to yourself

If you've just completed the *Every Man's Battle Workbook* on your own, and you found it to be a helpful and valuable experience, we encourage you to consider gathering a group of other men and helping lead them through this workbook together.

You'll find more information about starting a group on pages 236–37 of the section called Questions You May Have About This Workbook.

about the authors

STEPHEN ARTERBURN is founder and chairman of New Life Ministries and host of the nationally syndicated radio show, *New Life Live!* heard across the United States and on XM and Sirius satellite. Founder of the Women of Faith Conferences, he is a best-selling author and co-author of over seventy books including the Every Man and Every Woman series and his most recent book, *Being Christian*. He has been nominated for numerous writing awards and won three Gold Medallion awards for writing excellence, carries degrees from Baylor University and the University of North Texas, and obtained two honorary doctorate degrees. Steve resides with his family in Laguna Beach, California.

FRED STOEKER is a best-selling author of several books, including *Tactics* and *Hero,* the president of Living True Ministries, and a popular conference speaker who challenges men to become sexually pure, to reconnect in true intimate relationships with their wives, and to train their sons to become godly men. A graduate of Stanford University, Fred lives in Des Moines, Iowa, with his wife, Brenda, and their children.

MIKE YORKEY, a writer living in Encinitas, California, has collaborated with Fred Stoeker on all his books for the Every Man series.

Win the War on
Sexual Temptation at Every Age